Your Pregnancy Devotional

Your Pregnancy Devotional

280 Days of Prayer and Inspiration

Pamela Fierro and Suzie Chafin

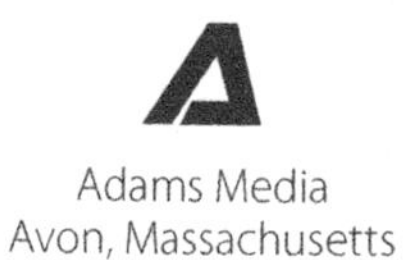

Adams Media
Avon, Massachusetts

Published by
Adams Media, an F+W Publications Company
57 Littlefield Street, Avon, MA 02322. U.S.A.
www.adamsmedia.com

ISBN 10: 1-59869-225-9
ISBN 13: 978-1-59869-225-9

Printed in the United States of America.

J I H G F E D C B A

Library of Congress Cataloging-in-Publication Data
is available from the publisher.

This book is available at quantity discounts for bulk purchases.
For information, please call 1-800-289-0963.

To our grandmothers,
Mary Belle Judd and Marjorie Storter Stokes.

—Suzie & Pam

CONTENTS

Acknowledgements

The authors would like to acknowledge the individuals who assisted them in bringing this work to fruition, including Barb Doyen and Meredith O'Hayre. In addition, they wish to thank their friends, family members, and sisters-in-Christ for their support and prayers, especially Jennifer Anderson, Leeann Niccolini, Cindy Mayfield, Lori Sakaab, Melissa Rothe, Dawn Colquhoun and Ann Aschenbrenner.

To Andy, Sam, Lauren, Jon, and James, thank you for giving me the time, support and prayers to complete this book.—Suzie

To Brian, Meredith, and Lauren, your patient and steadfast support of my endeavors is a true blessing. With love and thanks, Pam.

Finally and most importantly, we give thanks and praise to the One who inspires us, our Lord and Savior, Jesus Christ. We are grateful that He brought us together as friends and writing partners and wish for our work to glorify Him.

FIRST TRIMESTER

Blessed Beginnings

Introduction to the First Trimester

The first trimester of pregnancy is an exciting time. It's the beginning of your motherhood journey, and just like Genesis, the first book in the Bible, it starts with creation.

In the beginning there's just you. The first trimester actually begins before you're even pregnant. When defined as a forty-week period of gestation, the days of pregnancy start ticking about two weeks before conception, coinciding with your last menstrual period (LMP). About a week and a half after your period ends, your body prepares to ovulate. Hormones prompt your ovaries to release an egg, which travels down your Fallopian tube. If, perchance, the egg meets sperm and the conditions are right for conception, you're on your way to pregnancy!

The fusion of egg and sperm begins the journey toward the uterus. It's a microscopic organism, a pinpoint. Starting as a single cell, it begins a process of rapid cell division. A bubble grows around it, which will fill with fluid and form the amniotic sac. Frond-like wisps of tissue sprout forth, anchoring it to the soft lining of the uterus. About ten days after conception, the embryo implants in the uterus. Mom, you're officially pregnant!

Despite the furious activity being undertaken on the inside, you may or may not have any clue about your new status right away. But your body is changing, getting ready. Even before the embryo implants, it sends out chemical signals. Some of these chemicals are detectable in your urine, so when you take a pregnancy test, it will reveal the good news. As the weeks pass, your hormones trigger more changes throughout your body. Your uterus grows and expands to fill your pelvis, although it may not be visible through your abdomen yet. Nausea, dizziness, fatigue, and appetite changes are all common signs of pregnancy.

By the end of the first trimester, your baby has grown from a microscopic single-cell organism to a recognizably human form nearly four inches in size. The heart has formed and begun beating. Hands, fingers, legs, and toes are distinct. The eyes are nearly fully developed, although they remain fused shut for the time being. Though far from mature, all of the organs and systems that comprise your baby's physical structure are in place and beginning to function.

What a wondrous and amazing system God created for human reproduction! Although every life starts out in this same, seemingly simple way, the complex process of pregnancy—the creation of a new person—remains an astonishing and marvelous miracle.

DAY 1

Contemplating Conception

"See, I am sending an angel ahead of you to guard you along the way and to bring you to the place I have prepared."

EXODUS 23:20

Congratulations! You're on the path to motherhood. You've moved from "Someday we'll have a baby" to "I think we are ready." You're ready to enter a new phase in your family life. As a runner trains her body months before the big race, you have begun to physically and emotionally prepare yourself for the marathon of motherhood.

When the Israelites left Egypt to enter the Promised Land, they experienced daily miracles, witnessing firsthand God's generous provision for their every need. Yet, they grumbled and complained and even worshipped a golden calf. Though God had promised to go before them, giving them the ability to defeat their enemies, the Israelites were clouded with unbelief. When the time came to seize the Promised Land, they stood paralyzed, unable to move at God's command.

Unlike the Israelites, who heard the call yet were unbelieving, choose today to believe. God does what he says. Though the journey before you is uncharted and unknown to you, he will go before you, preparing the path, working behind the scenes, guarding and guiding you. †

DAY 2

Past, Present, Future

"Praise be to the God and Father of our LORD *Jesus Christ! In his great mercy he has given us new birth into a living hope through the resurrection of Jesus Christ from the dead. . . ."*

1 PETER 1:3

Do you know where you come from? The answer to that question has many facets: your genetic background, your family lineage, your hometown heritage. It's an important thing to contemplate as you consider your future as a parent.

Physically, your past may have relevance for your impending pregnancy and the children that you bear. One of the first things that a doctor or midwife will investigate is your medical history.

Isn't it nice to know that in Christ, you don't need a history? In Christ, you already have a full and complete identity. You have been rescued from the "dominion of darkness" (Colossians 1:13). You are "rooted" and growing in Christ (Colossians 2:7). You have been "raised with Christ" and "will appear with him in Glory" (Colossians 3:1–4).

You don't have to worry about what's in the past—the mistakes you've made years, months, or even hours ago—to have an identity in Christ. You are his child, a perfect creature; he calls you his own. †

DAY 3

The Spring

"For God, who said, 'Let light shine out of darkness,' made his light shine in our hearts to give us the light of the knowledge of the glory of God in the face of Christ."

2 CORINTHIANS 4:6

Every spring, I look forward to starting my garden. I love digging in the dirt; there is nothing like the feel of fresh soil between my fingers. I love the smell of the earth coming to life, the cultivating of the ground in preparation for growing. Gardening is so fulfilling—pulling weeds, planting seeds and flowers.

It always reminds me of how God prepares a mother's heart. First he takes fresh soil, preparing her heart for a baby. Then a seed is planted in her womb. She nurtures the baby growing inside her, giving it the light of her love, nourishing it with her own blood.

Do you feel like you need watering? Allow his Word to quench your thirst. Reading his Word brings you closer to Christ—radiance even when the world seems dark. His wisdom will illuminate your life if you let it. †

DAY 4

Egg Whites

"For the revelation awaits an appointed time; it speaks of the end and will not prove false. Though it linger, wait for it; it will certainly come and will not delay."

HABAKKUK 2:3

Who knew the term *egg whites* would take on such meaning when you're trying to conceive? The mysterious inner workings of your body are revealed with some interesting signs. You may be monitoring those signs, hoping to maximize your chances of conceiving soon. Between waiting for cervical mucus to be egg-white in consistency and watching basal temperature variations, you might feel like a giant science experiment.

Although you can do your part, ultimately your pregnancy is in God's hands. Assessing the signs and symptoms of your body's rhythms can help, but God's timing is perfect. The appropriate timing of conception is in his hands. †

Keep on Walkin'

"'. . . but let him who boasts boast about this: that he understands and knows me, that I am the LORD, *who exercises kindness, justice and righteousness on earth, for in these I delight,' declares the* LORD."

JEREMIAH 9:24

As you begin to plan for your pregnancy, these weeks are a great time to establish healthy habits and get your body in shape for the physical demands of an impending pregnancy. Physical exercise prepares your body, but what about exercising the spiritual "muscles" that God asks us to use, such as kindness, goodness, humility, and love? It's easy to slip up and not exercise the grace that God wants us to extend.

It's natural to focus inward before and during the pregnancy experience. So many wondrous things are occurring inside! So much is happening to you, and you are busy making exciting plans for your expanding family. However, God's Word reminds us that he delights in kindness, justice, and righteousness, qualities that require focus on others and not just on ourselves. †

DAY 6

Advanced Maternal Age

"Therefore, if anyone is in Christ, he is a new creation; the old has gone, the new has come! All this is from God, who reconciled us to himself through Christ and gave us the ministry of reconciliation: . . ."

2 CORINTHIANS 5:17–18

My sister-in-law became pregnant with her fourth child this past year. As a model, she is in an industry where age defines the success and duration of a career. However, she never thought her age would define her identity in motherhood. After her first doctor's visit, she was crowned with a new label: "Advanced Maternal Age." A woman at age thirty-five now feels as though she is deserving of geriatric prenatal care.

Isn't it wonderful that your identity in Christ has nothing to do with how old you are? He doesn't look at your age or beauty or other worldly markers for success. He sees you as his creation, the child he loves. Whether you are young or old, a first-time mom or a seasoned veteran, he has purposed you for motherhood in this season of your life. †

DAY 7

Horse Pills

". . . your eyes saw my unformed body. All the days ordained for me were written in your book before one of them came to be."

PSALM 139:16

You've been told those huge pills are supposedly vitamins. They look and smell terrible. When you choke them down, gulping a glass of water, they go down like horse pills. The throat constricts, resisting them. They cause nausea, and they back you up. Yet, each time you struggle to take one of these prenatal vitamins, remember why you are doing it. These vitamins are for the baby, the baby-to-be, the baby you hope God gives you.

When the day comes, you want your body to be in tip-top condition, physically ready to nourish your child. May each pill be a visual reminder of the goal in sight. Let it prompt prayer for the baby as you pause to take the vitamin each morning. You don't know when, who, or how, but the LORD does. He knows us before we are made, and we are his. †

DAY 8

More Than Me

"How great you are, O Sovereign LORD*! There is no one like you, and there is no God but you, as we have heard with our own ears."*

2 SAMUEL 7:22

With all of the planning, counting, calendar consulting, timing, temperature taking, book reading, buying of ovulation kits, monitoring, and (of course!) lovemaking, it's easy to forget that this baby is not about "me." This baby is not about what "I" want, what is best for "me," or what will make "me" happy. Does it really matter if the baby is scheduled before summer or after Christmas?

It's funny how we forget about the miracle of the child. We forget that babies are not about convenience or completing ourselves or trying to save a marriage or the ideal timing of maternity leave, but about a child—conceiving a new life to love, teach, and raise as a child of God. God has a purpose for this child that goes far beyond what will make "me" happy. When will this baby come? When God wants the baby to come. For what purpose? For his purpose. †

DAY 9

Little Things Mean a Lot

"For he will command his angels concerning you to guard you in all your ways; . . ."

PSALM 91:11

Small things make a big difference. Contemplating conception often prompts a woman to make small changes that could have a big impact on her child, like switching out the daily Starbucks fix to a vitamin-packed Jamba Juice, or choosing a glass of water rather than a glass of merlot with dinner. Taking a prenatal vitamin with folic acid can help eliminate the risk of possible birth defects of the brain or spine, a small choice that provides big results.

Like the pre-emptive protection your lifestyle changes provide for your baby, God rescues us from harm every day, surrounding us with angels to shield us. Usually, we can't even begin to grasp how God is working in our lives. It's the ringing cell phone that slows down a driver who is about to run a red light. Or the clearing of an otherwise busy road before a two-year-old darts into it. Sometimes it is just a stranger unknowingly speaking the right word of encouragement at the moment you need it most. These small miracles happen every day, all around us, a continual reminder of God working in our lives. †

DAY 10

Lingering Sadness

"He lifted me out of the slimy pit, out of the mud and mire; he set my feet on a rock and gave me a firm place to stand."

Psalm 40:2

After delivering two healthy, beautiful children, our friend felt like it was time to have another child. After months of pregnancy she lost the baby, filling her with grief and sadness. Soon, after receiving the doctor's permission, they tried again. After easily conceiving again, she miscarried once more.

They didn't understand what was happening, why God was allowing such heights of joy to be followed by such searing pain. After discovering the source of her body's difficulty in carrying a baby, they tried again. Now, two children later, the family knows the struggle was worth the reward.

Have you been through a miscarriage? It's hard to try again, knowing the pain you've endured in the past. Are you called to be a mother? If God has not removed that desire to conceive a child, try again. Life requires stepping out in faith, taking chances, living with faith. Don't let the pain of the past keep you from experiencing the hope of the future. †

DAY 11

Little Tricks

"Jesus looked at them and said, 'With man this is impossible, but with God all things are possible.'"

MATTHEW 19:26

There are all kinds of theories about how to improve your chances of conceiving. They range from the scientific to the superstitious, from eating wild yams to changing your underwear style to standing on your head. You might be tempted to try some of the suggestions you read online or tricks that your friends swear worked for them. It couldn't hurt, right?

Everything we try in our own power, though, is ultimately futile if it is not in God's timing. When we act in our own strength, assuming "we" can get the job done, we're not recognizing God's sovereignty. God is the central element of the conception equation. He has ordained the exact moment of conception in accordance with his plan for your family. †

DAY 12

Living Water

". . . Jesus stood and said in a loud voice, 'If anyone is thirsty, let him come to me and drink. Whoever believes in me, as the Scripture has said, streams of living water will flow from within him.'"

JOHN 7:37–38

You're not even pregnant yet, but do you find yourself constantly dashing to the bathroom? Perhaps it's due to drinking all of those glasses of water to keep yourself hydrated, creating the perfect environment for pregnancy to occur. Does this condition have you wondering what it will be like when you are actually pregnant and your bladder is compressed by a baby growing next to it?

Isn't it assuring to know that God is our perfect hydration? He is there, the living water, to refresh us when we are down, to restore us when we are broken, and to extend his mercy in our repentance. Thank you, God, for your never-ending supply of living water. It is there for the asking, paid for by Christ at the cross. †

Stuck in a Rut

"Let him kiss me with the kisses of his mouth—for your love is more delightful than wine."

SONG OF SONGS 1:2

Has your lovemaking transitioned from the passion of newlyweds to a prescription for inducing conception? Rather than spontaneous lovemaking, prompted by attraction or sexual tension, it seems like now it's reduced to "getting the job done."

Lovemaking is a gift from the Father to bring intimacy and unity to your relationship. God gave you this gift that transcends the reproductive purpose; it is your ability to commune together, allowing your bodies to express your love for one another without words. If lovemaking has become simply about getting pregnant, make a conscious choice to return to more meaningful lovemaking. Before you enter your marriage bed, desire your husband for who he is, not for the baby he can give you. ✝

DAY 14

Stomping Cigarettes

"Therefore put on the full armor of God, so that when the day of evil comes, you may be able to stand your ground, and after you have done everything, to stand."

EPHESIANS 6:13

When you see a smoker with a cigarette, do you have an uncontrollable urge to jerk it from his hands and stomp it out? Don't you want to shout, "Don't blow these pollutants on me!" You're not even pregnant yet, but just the possibility of carrying another life incites you to protect your baby at any cost. The maternal urge to protect a child is fiercely strong. It is being instilled in you even now, in the earliest days of motherhood.

Dangers will exist every day in this world: from environmental hazards to natural disasters to people who don't keep your child's best interests at heart. In every event, there will be circumstances that are completely out of your control. Isn't it comforting to know that your baby has God on her side? No matter what this world throws at your child, your baby has the Alpha and the Omega, the Creator and author of life, in her corner. There is no better place to be. †

DAY 15

Doesn't She Have Enough?

"Humble yourselves, therefore, under God's mighty hand, that he may lift you up in due time. Cast all your anxiety on him because he cares for you."

1 PETER 5:6–7

Have you ever walked by a woman who seemingly had a truckload of kids? You hear them coming before they even get out of the car. As she emerges, you catch a glimpse of her swollen belly, thinking, "What does that make it? Like, baby number eight?"

Your eyes glance down at your own flat belly, still the same as yesterday. "Why is it so easy for some, God, while others require so much waiting?" Wait on him. He will lift you up in due time. We never know why God has said "not now" or "just wait." He has an answer for your prayer, though it seems to make no sense to you now. His answer—in accordance with his perfect plan for your life—will reveal itself in his time. †

DAY 16

Was Last Night THE Night?

". . . guide me in your truth and teach me, for you are God my Savior, and my hope is in you all day long."

PSALM 25:5

Have you felt a quickening in your spirit, a sign that perhaps you've conceived? Maybe you had a special night with your husband; it felt like it was THE night. When I was first pregnant with my first child, I was in church, in the middle of praising God, and I just sensed it.

Do you have a sense in your spirit that you could be pregnant? Perhaps you're trying to ignore your suspicion, afraid that you're setting yourself up for another month of disappointment. The pain of disappointment is sharp, especially if you've experienced it in months past.

Is it false hope? Possibly, but it is also possible that your hunch is correct. No matter what this month means, what is revealed in the days ahead, you still have hope in Christ. When we choose to hope in him, we will always be satisfied, fulfilled, and at peace. His hope is eternal, everlasting. Hope in him. †

DAY 17

New Thoughts

"'For I know the plans I have for you,' declares the LORD, *'plans to prosper you and not to harm you, plans to give you hope and a future.'"*

JEREMIAH 29:11

Are you tired of thinking about getting pregnant? Do you feel like too many hours of your day are spent waiting and wondering, praying for pregnancy? Is your mind wandering, unable to focus on anything except the possibility of secret activity deep inside your womb? Do you find yourself releasing your anxiety and expectation for pregnancy to God, only to take it back again moments later with the newest pang of worry?

Give it to him entirely. Trust God's Word with full confidence, standing on his promise. Release your worry and any anxiety and focus on new thoughts. God's purpose is to give you a future and hope, not to keep you in a state of suspension. When your mind starts to wander, fill it with his Word by repeating his promise. "I know the plans I have for you . . . plans to prosper you and not to harm you, plans to give you hope and a future." †

DAY 18

The Waiting Game

"I wait for the LORD, *my soul waits, and in his word I put my hope."*

PSALM 130:5

Wouldn't the waiting be easier if you already knew the answer? If you knew by a certain date that you'd have a baby, would it make the waiting game easier? No one really knows what the future holds, not fortune tellers or prognosticators or even the *National Enquirer*.

Do you want this baby so much that you can almost feel him in your arms? Do you visualize yourself pushing the stroller, carrying the diaper bag, showing off your baby to admiring friends and family? Be sure that it is not just the illusion of motherhood that you've fallen in love with. Rather, focus your thoughts today on waiting on God, first seeking God's will for your life.

Motherhood is a chance to impact, shape, and love another life. Take a moment today to read about other women who waited for God's timing in conceiving a child: Abraham's wife, Sarah (Genesis 21), Hannah (1 Samuel 1), and Rachel (Genesis 30:22–24). God has preserved their stories just for you so that you can learn his lessons through them. Instead of putting your hope in the things of this world—a stroller or a crib—put your hope in his Word. †

DAY 19

Just in Case

"Therefore, since we are surrounded by such a great cloud of witnesses, let us throw off everything that hinders and the sin that so easily entangles, and let us run with perseverance the race marked out for us. Let us fix our eyes on Jesus, the author and perfecter of our faith, who for the joy set before him endured the cross, scorning its shame, and sat down at the right hand of the throne of God. Consider him who endured such opposition from sinful men, so that you will not grow weary and lose heart."

HEBREWS 12:1–3

There it sits, nestled in your bathroom cabinet, between the bars of soap, shampoo bottles, and toilet paper rolls. The box has been shaken, looked at, opened, and explored. The directions to the test have been read and reread, to ensure future accuracy. You hold it, wondering, "What will it say?" One day quite soon, you'll take the pregnancy test and watch for its results. Will the symbol it reveals make you laugh and smile, crying tears of joy? Or will the answer cause you to cry in frustration, another symbol of delay and waiting?

The symbol on the pregnancy test is not what matters though. Hope is not found in a positive pregnancy test. Real hope is found at the cross where Jesus Christ conquered sin. Look to the cross this week for your symbol of him, the one who has his loving arms wrapped tightly around you, carrying you through these weeks. †

DAY 20

The Pillow

"Now to him who is able to do immeasurably more than all we ask or imagine, according to his power that is at work within us, to him be glory in the church and in Christ Jesus throughout all generations, for ever and ever!"

EPHESIANS 3:20–21

Every woman probably does it sometime. Maybe you've done it too. Did you use one or two pillows, stuffing them inside your shirt, pulling your shirt back to reveal what you will look like pregnant? For a moment you get a glimpse, a future picture of what you might look like in a few months. Caressing your growing belly, you imagine the baby growing inside you.

Your daydream comes to an abrupt halt, right as you remember that you were eight years old the last time you played this imagination game. God's ability to work in us goes so far beyond our imagination. No matter where you are today—whatever you look like, whether you are a mother or a daughter, a sister or a friend—in him, you are a creation that he loves and adores. You are his. †

DAY 21

Swollen Skin

"I am not saying this because I am in need, for I have learned to be content whatever the circumstances. I know what it is to be in need, and I know what it is to have plenty. I have learned the secret of being content in any and every situation, whether well fed or hungry, whether living in plenty or in want. I can do everything through him who gives me strength."

PHILIPPIANS 4:11–13

Everywhere you look, there are visual reminders of what you don't have: your friend's bulging belly, the cute clothes in the maternity store, mothers pushing strollers, and pictures of cherubic infants smiling in magazine ads. Do you feel like crying out, "What about me? When is it my turn?" Do you long to rub your own swollen skin, to feel the baby within?

It's easy to feel itchy and antsy, eager for the future to be revealed and anxious to get to the next stage of your motherhood. It's human nature to be driven by what our eyes see of our circumstances, to covet for ourselves what we see in those around us. It's much more difficult to let God's nature fill our hearts with contentment and acceptance.

God has put you where you are today for a purpose. Be content where you are for this moment. These days of preparation and waiting are not without purpose, and he can make today full. He has promised to supply all your needs (Philippians 4:19), and for today, allow that promise to make you full, pleased, and content. †

DAY 22

The Apple of His Eye

"In a desert land he found him, in a barren and howling waste. He shielded him and cared for him; he guarded him as the apple of his eye. . . ."

DEUTERONOMY 32:10

It can be bittersweet, holding a baby when your heart longs for one of your own. You help the mom change the baby's diaper, count the tiny toes, let the little hand wrap around your finger. As you watch another's child being cradled, loved, rocked, and nurtured, God reminds you that he is holding you. God knows the desire of your heart; he knows exactly what you want.

He is holding you, as a father holds his own baby, whispering a sweet "Shhhh" in your ear. Just as the new father is proud, with his protective arms wrapped around the apple of his eye, so is your heavenly Father proud of you. Deuteronomy 32:11 illustrates God's protection as "like an eagle that stirs up its nest and hovers over its young, that spread its wings to catch them and carries them on its pinions." He feels the same way about you. He will shield you and care for you, even when you find yourself in a "desert land" of worry or hurt. †

DAY 23

PMS or Pregnancy?

"What you heard from me, keep as the pattern of sound teaching, with faith and love in Christ Jesus. Guard the good deposit that was entrusted to you—guard it with the help of the Holy Spirit who lives in us."

2 TIMOTHY 1:13–14

One thing I did know was that I didn't feel well. My head hurt, my breasts were sore, and cramps—oh, the cramps. They just wouldn't go away. A day passed and no period. Two days passed and I called my girlfriend. "It's probably just PMS," she soothed. Yes, yes, of course, she was right. Why would I be feeling cramps if I am pregnant? Don't you get a respite from those PMS symptoms if you're pregnant?

Another day passed and then another. "Should I take a test?" I wondered. Should I just figure it out somehow? Is it too early to know for sure? Will I jinx myself if I act too soon?

Our symptoms for one thing are also symptoms for another. So it's hard to know when the aches and discomfort are associated with PMS or pregnancy. What we do know is that God has left us his deposit, as a pledge guaranteeing our future inheritance (Ephesians 1:13–14). The Holy Spirit is our constant companion. We know that this heavenly deposit is all we need. †

DAY 24

Choices, Choices

"And pray in the Spirit on all occasions with all kinds of prayers and requests. With this in mind, be alert and always keep on praying for all the saints."

EPHESIANS 6:18

The shelf in the drugstore displaying pregnancy tests has more choices than the grocery store has types of peanut butter. Which one, God? Which one is the most accurate? Do I need two? If I am pregnant, isn't one enough? But then what if I do it wrong or I can't read the results?

Before you know it, your shopping basket is full of pregnancy test kits. It may feel silly, asking God to help you with the right pregnancy test. Does he care about such things? Yes, absolutely. I used to think I should "save" my requests to God, as if there were a limited supply. Once I hit a certain number, his ear would go deaf, so I'd better prioritize my prayers and send up only the biggest petitions.

Now I know that God wants us to come to him with all of those small details—even the littlest things—not just the big problems. Our prayer life should resemble a constant conversation, ongoing all day long, as we talk to him about everything. †

DAY 25

Quasi-Pregnant?

"Yet to all who received him, to those who believed in his name, he gave the right to become children of God. . . ."

JOHN 1:12

I went to the doctor to have a blood test. The pregnancy test kit from the drugstore said yes, but I needed medical confirmation. Was I really pregnant? The doctor's answer was, "Yes, but come back tomorrow for another test."

What? Why? They needed to make sure that the HCG levels in my blood had doubled. So I went back the next day, and the next. Meanwhile, I wasn't sure what it meant. I felt like I was in this pregnancy limbo, that I was only pregnant for that day, because tomorrow's test might prove otherwise.

Finally, my HCG level rose to a place where I was confident enough to call myself pregnant. Thankfully, in Christ, there is no minimum level, no temporary sense of limbo. We are either in Christ or not. We can't drop below a minimum standard or suddenly become so ugly or so sinful that he would not love us anymore. Through Christ, we have received complete reconciliation. Thank you, God, for loving me where I am today. †

DAY 26

Was That the Starting Gun?

"This is what the Lord *says—your Redeemer, the Holy One of Israel: 'I am the* Lord *your God, who teaches you what is best for you, who directs you in the way you should go.'"*

Isaiah 48:17

Do you sit, wondering, "Am I really pregnant, God? Really, really, really?"

As the reality of pregnancy settles in, you may have mixed feelings. Are you torn between jumping up and down in delight and falling to your knees, realizing life will never be the same again?

A new path has begun. You're standing at the starting line of a great race, and the gun has just gone off. Your feet are moving, you have started the race down the path of pregnancy, but it all still feels a bit surreal.

Don't worry, God is with you. Every time you face a fear or a worry, as a child of God, you have the right to approach the throne of grace to find his mercy in your time of need (Hebrews 4:16). You have a Father who will be with you step by step, moment by moment, in every way, every day. He'll run the race with you, through each doctor appointment, through each pang of worry, through all of your body's changes. †

DAY 27

Copilot

"The Lord *is my strength and my song; he has become my salvation. He is my God, and I will praise him, my father's God, and I will exalt him."*

Exodus 15:2

Despite all of your physical and emotional preparation for pregnancy, when it actually happens, you realize quite clearly how little control you actually have. From the moment that sperm meets egg, the events occurring in your body are not within your command. The journey to your uterus, the implantation in your womb, and the infinite division and development of tiny cells are happening under the guidance of a higher authority. Will it be a girl? A boy? Twins? Will this baby have blond hair? His father's dimples? Her mother's eyes? These aren't options you can select from a program.

It's as though God has asked you to copilot this most important flight. He is holding the controls, but you're asked to come alongside on the journey, doing what he asks, responding to his requests. To be an efficient copilot, you must trust your pilot implicitly and remain in constant communication. Trust God, your pilot, with ultimate control of your pregnancy journey. †

DAY 28

Just Slipped

". . . neither height nor depth, nor anything else in all creation, will be able to separate us from the love of God that is in Christ Jesus our LORD."

ROMANS 8:39

I had these great plans of surprising him with the news. I racked my brain for original, clever ways to tell my husband that he was going to be a father. My friends shared all kinds of cute stories, and I wanted my news to be as creative and inspired as a marriage proposal.

Yet, when it came down to it, my cleverness and wit evaporated; the joy was too great. I couldn't contain myself; the news just slipped out. Isn't that the way that God feels about us? He doesn't just tolerate us. Rather, he loves us passionately; he enjoys us. He desires a relationship with us. The way he loves us is too great to contain, too vast to measure. Thank you, God, for loving us so. †

DAY 29

Freeze Tag

"'Listen to this, Job; stop and consider God's wonders. Do you know how God controls the clouds and makes his lightning flash? Do you know how the clouds hang poised, those wonders of him who is perfect in knowledge?'"

JOB 37:14–16

Do you feel like someone has tagged you in a game of freeze tag? Now that you realize you are pregnant, do you feel frozen, afraid to move? You don't want to do anything that could potentially jeopardize your baby's health. Everything seems to be harmful: from exercise to food to the very air you breathe. How easily your fear can steal your joy.

Even though the world seems full of harm, rest assured that God is in control. Though you get to make the choices about what you eat and how you take care of your body, you simply can't guard against every possible pitfall, and you don't have to. In Isaiah 41:10, God says to each of us, "So do not fear, for I am with you; do not be dismayed, for I am your God. I will strengthen you and help you; I will uphold you with my righteous right hand." Don't remain frozen by fear, but face each day boldly, knowing your God is strengthening and helping you, holding you with his hand. †

DAY 30

My Mouth Hurts

"My lips will shout for joy when I sing praise to you—I, whom you have redeemed."

PSALM 71:23

The symptoms of pregnancy take some odd forms. Personally, I never really felt like I had the special "glow" attributed to pregnancy. My nails were only marginally stronger, and my hair never seemed to take on the luster described in all of the books. What I did notice was that my cheeks and mouth hurt all the time. I would feel them hurting, unsure of the cause, and then realize I was doing it again: smiling.

I'd rub them out only to feel them sore again. I just could not stop smiling at the thought of the life growing inside of me. Of all the symptoms I read about pregnancy, uncontrollable smiling never made the list, yet the joy I felt was undeniable. Our new life in Christ can produce joy as well, true joy that transcends any circumstance in life. It is the kind of joy that is not dependent upon success, failure, health, or sickness. Thank you, God, for the joy you give me. †

DAY 31

A Hidden Place

"They will speak of the glorious splendor of your majesty, and I will meditate on your wonderful works. They will tell of the power of your awesome works, and I will proclaim your great deeds."

PSALM 145:5–6

Somewhere, hidden deep within your body, is a secret place. You can't see it or touch it, and even if you could, you probably wouldn't recognize anything humanly familiar. Inside that hidden place, a miracle is happening. A life is growing, moment by moment. Though only millimeters in size, your baby is being carefully crafted, knit together in your womb. It's just the beginning of your pregnancy, yet you are already filled with such love for this little life. Each day as the child grows, amazingly so will your love.

God is at work in every moment and in every detail. He is carefully weaving together the cells that will compose your child's limbs, organs, and brain. God is grafting your child together, instilling talents, hair color, strengths, and abilities. How awesome you are, God! †

DAY 32

Give Me a Job!

"It is the Lord *your God you must follow, and him you must revere. Keep his commands and obey him; serve him and hold fast to him."*

Deuteronomy 13:4

During these early days of pregnancy, you're trying to give your baby the best start. Are you feeling like you want to do something more to help things along? Do you feel like shouting, "What else can I do?" So much of motherhood is about doing—caring, giving, feeding, clothing, cleaning up. Yet, for this part of pregnancy, you are called only to serve as the vessel God is using to grow this baby. Right now, it's not up to you to "do," but rather to "be."

Your role is central to the successful outcome of this pregnancy. Your participation in obtaining proper nutrition, exercise, and prenatal care is paramount. God has chosen you to help participate in the miracle of motherhood. Yet, the miracle is all his. Follow his instruction; obey his voice while walking in his will. When you are in his will, everything else has a way of working out. Your job is to remain there. †

DAY 33

A Beating Heart

"Love the LORD *your God with all your heart and with all your soul and with all your strength."*

DEUTERONOMY 6:5

Already, your child has acquired a heartbeat. His little heart will continue to grow into a full four-chambered organ, responsible for sustaining his circulation throughout his lifetime. A mere five weeks ago you were praying for this child who was not yet known, and now this baby has a heart that beats!

As a mother, you are dually concerned about your child's heart. Now, you want the baby's heart to grow physically, developing without defect or flaw. After your baby is born into this world, you'll never stop praying for his heart, the spiritual heart that will one day house the Holy Spirit. What kind of dwelling place will it be? Pray today that God would set the rhythm for your child's heartbeat. †

DAY 34

Gearing Up

"David said to the Philistine, 'You come against me with sword and spear and javelin, but I come against you in the name of the LORD *Almighty, the God of the armies of Israel, whom you have defied.'"*

1 SAMUEL 17:45

There are a lot of checklists associated with having a baby. Vitamins, doctors, midwives, and doulas. Check. Pregnancy books, Internet sites, parenting magazines, and friends' advice. Check. Regular clothes, baggy clothes, maternity clothes (even though you don't need them yet!). Check.

With so much preparation under way for this little life, it almost feels like a soldier who is gearing up for battle. It's easy to physically prepare for a baby, but preparing your spirit for motherhood is a different matter altogether. As you begin to prepare your body and prepare your home, remember to also take time to prepare your spirit. Spend time each day in God's Word. Give him the chance to whisper in your ear and stir your spirit. †

DAY 35

The Great Mothers

"My son, do not forget my teaching, but keep my commands in your heart, for they will prolong your life many years and bring you prosperity."

PROVERBS 3:1–2

The Bible provides some great examples of mothers. Take Mary, so favored by God that she was chosen to become the mother of Christ. Or Sarah, who waited faithfully for decades before giving birth to Isaac. Do you ever read about the great mothers in the Bible—Mary, Sarah, Elizabeth, Ruth, Hannah—and think, "I can never be like them"? Reading about their faith and greatness of character can make you feel inadequate, like you don't measure up.

Don't compare yourself unfavorably to these biblical mothers. Instead, savor their stories for the spiritual encouragement they provide. You don't have to have a fancy "title" or be an icon of this world to bear the title of "mother." Regardless of fame, fortune, status, or caliber, you are this child's mother and have the ability to impact, shape, and mold this life. What higher calling could there be? †

DAY 36

Christmas Eve

"Brothers, as an example of patience in the face of suffering, take the prophets who spoke in the name of the LORD. *As you know, we consider blessed those who have persevered. You have heard of Job's perseverance and have seen what the* LORD *finally brought about. The* LORD *is full of compassion and mercy."*

JAMES 5:10–11

Do you remember what it felt like to be a young child on Christmas Eve? The night seemed to stretch out endlessly; the hours passed slowly. Sleep was fitful, as you woke up to check the clock and to peek out the window in hopes of catching a glimpse of a sleigh or a reindeer. After a seeming eternity, the morning light would eventually come, the cue that it was safe to venture to the tree and see what magical transformation had occurred overnight.

Sometimes pregnancy feels like nine months of Christmas Eve. Rather than having to wait one night, you're facing thirty-five weeks of giddy anticipation, looking forward to the magical gift of a baby in your arms. When it feels like the time will never pass, call on the LORD to instill patience, allowing the weeks of waiting to only increase your joy in many tomorrows. †

DAY 37

It's a Date!

"Because of your great compassion you did not abandon them in the desert. By day the pillar of cloud did not cease to guide them on their path, nor the pillar of fire by night to shine on the way they were to take."

NEHEMIAH 9:19

It's official! Even though you may have known you were pregnant for some time now, there is something about that first prenatal visit that makes it feel official and certifiable. For one thing, you are given an estimated due date, an actual day that you can point to on a calendar. You can look at the months ahead and visualize the transition between pregnancy and motherhood.

You get to ask questions and talk about the baby with a doctor or midwife who is invested in caring for you and your baby. Do you feel God's hand on you as well? He's there too, alongside you and your medical caregiver, directing, guiding, and watching. God directed the Israelites in the desert, providing them direction by day and night, and he will do the same for you. †

DAY 38

Chosen One

"You did not choose me, but I chose you and appointed you to go and bear fruit—fruit that will last. Then the Father will give you whatever you ask in my name."

JOHN 15:16

I kept thinking, "Did you really choose me? Am I really able to raise a baby the way you want me to, God?" But he chose me just as he chose you. God requires faith in response to his call. Doubting, wondering, and second-guessing is of no benefit to anyone. In the first chapter of Luke, when an angel told Zechariah that his wife, Elizabeth, would bear a son, he doubted the angel's words. The angel Gabriel responded, "I am Gabriel. I stand in the presence of God, and I have been sent to speak to you and to tell you this good news. And now you will be silent and not able to speak until the day this happens, because you did not believe my words, which will come true at their proper time."

The LORD has chosen you to bear fruit by raising a child. God's promises command faith. Have the faith to know that God will meet you every day, wherever you are, enabling you to raise this child he has entrusted to you. †

DAY 39

Oh the Odors!

"He has filled the hungry with good things. . . ."

Luke 1:53

It happens overnight. One day you can open the refrigerator, ready to devour anything inside. The next, just the vapors from an onion in a plastic bag and the sight of the chicken from last night's dinner make your knees go weak. The thought of tuna fish sandwiches, which you found delicious a week ago, makes you begin to retch.

Morning sickness is an outward symptom and sign of the life growing within you. It can hijack your appetite in the morning, afternoon, evening, or even all day long. You aren't hungering for very much right now, so allow this time to be filled with hunger for the Lord. When odors turn your stomach, turn to God's Word. †

DAY 40

The Right Words

"When words are many, sin is not absent, but he who holds his tongue is wise."

PROVERBS 10:19

I didn't recognize the words coming out of my mouth, or the emotions raging inside of me. My husband didn't know whether to sit still or to try to speak. Either way it didn't matter; no matter what he did, it wouldn't be the right thing. It couldn't be the right thing, because I didn't even know what it was I wanted him to say or do.

It's hard for a husband to sit and watch the hormones and sickness ravage his wife. He wants to help but doesn't know how. You want him to help and are angry that he doesn't have an innate sense directing him how.

It's easy to let those angry little words slide off your tongue, but rein them in. Chances are you really don't even mean most of what you say, but that the hormones have taken control. Some moments it may be better to say nothing at all. †

DAY 41

Got Blessings?

"Praise be to the God and Father of our Lord *Jesus Christ, who has blessed us in the heavenly realms with every spiritual blessing in Christ."*

Ephesians 1:3

What are your thoughts fixed on? It's easy to dwell on what could go wrong in pregnancy and what you'll have to give up once you have this baby. There are so many worries and what-ifs, that you could drown in your concerns.

When those waves of worry start to crash over your head, it's time to count your blessings. Just close your eyes, breathe in and out, and think on him, deliberately refocusing your thoughts. What has God done for you lately? How has he answered prayer in your life? What are you thankful for in this moment? Every time you count your blessings, you come away reassured and relaxed. He has blessed you beyond measure, and one of his blessings is tucked safely inside of you. Praise him for his goodness. †

DAY 42

Out of Sync

"No temptation has seized you except what is common to man. And God is faithful; he will not let you be tempted beyond what you can bear. But when you are tempted, he will also provide a way out so that you can stand up under it."

1 CORINTHIANS 10:13

When you're pregnant, everything feels out of sync. When you stand up you feel like you need to sit down, yet sitting brings no relief either. You're starving, but you can't stand the sight or smell of food. If there is an upside to this fatigue and nausea, it is that temptations that might be hard to resist otherwise have absolutely no hold on you right now.

During these critical days of your baby's formation, you don't have to worry about resisting caffeine, because the thought of coffee makes you squirm. Nor would you consider fast food a delight, because the only thing that is palatable is saltine crackers. God always provides a way out of temptation! †

DAY 43

Shock Absorbers

"I lift up my eyes to the hills—where does my help come from? My help comes from the Lord, *the Maker of heaven and earth."*

Psalm 121:1–2

Your body is providing a safe growing place for your baby. Your uterus and the amniotic sac that cushion the baby serve as shock absorbers. They soften the impact of daily life, protecting and covering the baby so that, by the time it reaches him, what started out as a big jolt is a small ripple. The baby goes nowhere without you. Wherever you are, the baby will be.

God does that for us, too. He is omnipresent. He does not simply float in and out of our lives, waiting to make an appearance. He is consistently and always present, in every location, in every moment in the entire universe. Because of him, your life is lived much like the baby's inside your womb is. He is the shock absorber, smoothing out the big jolts in your life. Why? Because he loves you; you are his child that he is carrying. He loves you more than you can imagine. †

Prayer Warrior

"'Call to me and I will answer you and tell you great and unsearchable things you do not know.'"

JEREMIAH 33:3

My best friend, Angie, often tells of how she would find her mother on her knees every day. Her mother, so involved in praying for each of her three daughters, would be oblivious to her young daughter's presence. Angie would stand there, watching her mother actively seeking intercession for her family through prayer.

Now, as a mother of three children, Angie still leans on her mother's prayers. When she asks for prayer on her family's behalf, she knows with full confidence that her mother will willingly and eagerly seek God for them.

What an amazing example of God's love she is to her daughters. That is the kind of mother I want to be. I want my kids to see me on my knees, to know that in the middle of everything I can go to him and he will hear my prayers. Pray today that you will always be your child's prayer warrior. †

DAY 45

The Porcelain Throne

"Be on your guard; stand firm in the faith; be men of courage; be strong."

1 CORINTHIANS 16:13

When pregnant with my twins, I never expected to develop such a close relationship with our toilet bowl. My face was never meant to spend so much time peering inside it! No matter how many breath mints I sucked on, how many crackers I ate, or how much Sprite I sipped, that constant sick feeling just would not go away. While some things provided brief, temporary relief, what helped one day would send me straight to the bathroom the next.

But God was my healer. Morning sickness is a phase. A phase that seems like it will never end, but it does, little by little, in increments that finally leave you feeling like your old self. Time in that toilet seat was part of the process to bring about the end reward. Every moment spent there was worth it. †

DAY 46

Not a Zit!

"I do not understand what I do. For what I want to do I do not do, but what I hate I do. And if I do what I do not want to do, I agree that the law is good. As it is, it is no longer I myself who do it, but it is sin living in me. I know that nothing good lives in me, that is, in my sinful nature. For I have the desire to do what is good, but I cannot carry it out. For what I do is not the good I want to do; no, the evil I do not want to do—this I keep on doing. Now if I do what I do not want to do, it is no longer I who do it, but it is sin living in me that does it."

ROMANS 7:15–20

What is that on my chin? Could it be a pimple? Everyone wants a healthy pregnancy glow, not a full-blown breakout, reminiscent of teenage acne. It's bad enough that these hormones declare mutiny on your emotions, but on your face, too? It's so ugly, out there in plain sight for everyone to see!

What about you is ugly in God's sight? It's not what's plain on your face—not your skin, your hair, or your expanded belly. What kind of a breakout does God see in your character? Pray that he would reveal to you the sin in your life that is rearing its ugly head. Seek his guidance in clearing out those blemishes and flaws that are outside of his will. †

DAY 47

My Other Half

"My dove in the clefts of the rock, in the hiding places on the mountainside, show me your face, let me hear your voice; for your voice is sweet, and your face is lovely."

SONG OF SONGS 2:14

Is something coming between you and your husband—a little something called pregnancy? You may be spending a lot of your time and energy focusing on it instead of him. If you're not daydreaming about the baby, you're moping about your skin breaking out or your pants feeling tight. If you're not rushing to the bathroom, you're falling asleep before suppertime.

How can you reconnect with him this week? How can the two of you find a way to discover this new life together? Pregnancy can be a time when the two of you grow closer, tied together by the bond that is growing within you. Or, it can be the start of a subtle separateness, drawing you apart. Make the decision that this will not be a time to divide, to seek separate space and isolation, but a time that you choose to experience together. Show him that you still love him, adore him, and desire him. †

DAY 48

Ready to Listen?

"But if from there you seek the LORD *your God, you will find him if you look for him with all your heart and with all your soul."*

DEUTERONOMY 4:29

During pregnancy you'll find a long checklist of what you should and shouldn't do: eat this, don't eat that, stay hydrated, take vitamins, exercise, avoid toxins, get plenty of rest. Yet all of the advice and guidelines mean nothing if the words of instruction are not followed. A pregnant woman who chooses to ignore the recommendations can put herself and her baby in jeopardy.

In your spiritual walk, you have also been given orders. God expects you to follow his will and heed his laws. He also provides plenty of resources to help you along the way, from friends to hold you accountable, to the Holy Spirit, guiding from within. You also have the perfect example of Christ, who intercedes for you even when you falter. And when you need specific instruction, you can always turn to the Bible to clarify your concerns, questions, needs, and doubts.

As in pregnancy, if you don't listen to and heed the advice, you put yourself at risk. Are you ready to listen? †

Fingers and Toes

"'I am with you and will watch over you wherever you go, and I will bring you back to this land. I will not leave you until I have done what I have promised you.'"

Genesis 28:15

Do you wish you could peek inside your belly? What would you see? Although far from resembling the baby you will take home from the hospital, certain familiar characteristics are starting to form. Baby is starting to develop fingers and toes. Where will those fingers and toes carry him or her? What kind of journey does God have for this baby?

It's exciting—and sometimes a little bit scary—to think about the future potential for the tiny life that is just beginning to develop. You want your child to have a well-lived life, but not to experience pain. You want your child to have everything you can give her, but not to be spoiled. What will this child's journey be? What plans do you have for her? The one constant throughout her life will be her heavenly Father. From this moment until the moment of Glory, God will be with her. †

DAY 50

Oranges

"You are my hiding place; you will protect me from trouble and surround me with songs of deliverance. Selah"

PSALM 32:7

Next time you are in the supermarket, pick up an orange. Hold it next to your tummy. Can you visualize the size of your uterus better now? Tucked away safely inside your orange-sized uterus is your child. (You might see the watermelons nearby and start thinking ahead. Whoa! Let's just focus on today.) Hold on to that little orange, a visual reminder of the hiding place your child occupies in your womb.

As a child my hiding place was in my closet, where I'd outfitted a small refuge. I'd go there to cry when I was sad, read with a flashlight when I wanted privacy, or just sit quietly when I needed time to think.

Though life is busier today (and my children would surely follow me into my closet if I tried to escape there!), I still need a hiding place, a moment in time to give praises to God and refresh my spirit. No matter where we are, whether in a crowded room or alone in an isolated place, God is always our hiding place. In him we have refuge. †

DAY 51

Scales and Measures

"He humbled you, causing you to hunger and then feeding you with manna, which neither you nor your fathers had known, to teach you that man does not live on bread alone but on every word that comes from the mouth of the LORD.*"*

DEUTERONOMY 8:3

What is your relationship with the scale? Do you greet it enthusiastically each day, eager to see the numbers increasing as proof of your pregnant progression? Or do you ignore it, deliberately passing it by, thinking, "I don't really need to know the answer to that question."

Just as you go to God and entrust him with your baby's health, go to him with yours. Ask him to help you control your urges and cravings. Ask him to help you make wise choices, giving you the strength to eat healthy, nourishing food.

God's power is beyond limit. It can't be weighed or measured. You have access to that power through the Holy Spirit, which becomes a part of you when you accept Christ as your savior. Why get bogged down by numbers on a scale when your true worth is measured by Christ's love? †

DAY 52

Hurting Head

"Have mercy on me, O God, have mercy on me, for in you my soul takes refuge. I will take refuge in the shadow of your wings until the disaster has passed."

PSALM 57:1

Every time I was pregnant, I was plagued with headaches throughout the entire first trimester. My headaches were horrible, pounding events, making it impossible even to run a simple errand. I could not understand how my child, something just the size of a grain of rice growing inside of something the size of an orange, could turn my body so completely upside down.

It's easy to focus on pain or discomfort when it is all we can feel at the moment. Yet pain—all pain—is temporal and serves a purpose. It alerts us of injury, and encourages us to slow down or to seek medical care. Emotional pain causes us to cling to God, to realize that we can't live this life on our own, and to discover a new sense of compassion and empathy with others. No one likes to live in discomfort, but trust God with your pain. He will use it for his glory. †

DAY 53

Eating for Two?

"Do you not know that your body is a temple of the Holy Spirit, who is in you, whom you have received from God? You are not your own; you were bought at a price. Therefore honor God with your body."

1 CORINTHIANS 6:19–20

Is eating for two a mission or a myth about pregnancy? Is it truly an accurate statement? During pregnancy, I liked to think it was true—I didn't harbor as much guilt when I justified my junk-food binges as eating for two. But does a half-inch-long baby really need as much nourishment as a full-grown woman does?

The Word instructs us that our bodies are as temples. Consider how you would treat your church. You would never bring anything offensive into your sanctuary—whether through word or deed. Yet, when we choose to make unhealthy eating choices, we are offending and misusing our bodies, the personal temple God has given us. During pregnancy, eating wisely means eating proportionately. Eat more healthy foods more often. For now, consider instead that you are really eating for one—your baby. You are God's vessel and the choices you make should glorify him. †

DAY 54

Feeling Down?

"Restore to me the joy of your salvation and grant me a willing spirit, to sustain me."

PSALM 51:12

Some days you just drag. You can't explain it, and you know that if you wait a day or so it will pass. Your body is weary, your thoughts are unfocused. You don't know why the sky seems dull, or why you don't feel like talking to anyone. There are some days when you just feel like sleeping instead of living.

Everyone needs to be revived from time to time. Are you in the doldrums? If you need a little pick-me-up, something to make you smile, dig into God's Word. Open up your Bible and see how he speaks to you today. Will the praises of the Psalms infuse your joy? Will the good news of the Gospel restore your hope? Just like a cool rain will revive a plant after a drought, God's Word can revive your spirit when you're feeling low. †

DAY 55

He Is Proud

"The man with the two talents also came. 'Master,' he said, 'you entrusted me with two talents; see, I have gained two more.' His master replied, 'Well done, good and faithful servant! You have been faithful with a few things; I will put you in charge of many things. Come and share your master's happiness!'"

MATTHEW 25:22–23

A child yearns to hear the words "I'm proud of you" from her parents. It is validation that she is loved, that she is doing what her parents desire. Hearing those words can inspire a child to soar in life. Do you ever wonder if your heavenly Father is proud of you? You might think, "I know I'm forgiven, but have I made him proud?"

He doesn't view success as the world does. Fancy titles, wealth, and possessions don't impress God. What makes him proud is how you serve him each day, how you glorify him through what you say and do. Every time you show love to a stranger or defend his name, you make him proud. Every time you use one of the gifts he has given you, he is proud. Though everyone gets off track and makes bad choices from time to time, his grace ensures that you can return to a closer walk with him and make him proud again. †

DAY 56

Droopy Lids

"Be at rest once more, O my soul, for the LORD *has been good to you."*

PSALM 116:7

Oh, the fatigue of these early weeks of pregnancy. Do you feel like you need to take a nap just to recover from waking up and rising out of bed? With your job and family responsibilities, you may feel like you don't have time to be tired. But God has ways of slowing us down. The feelings of fatigue are God's reminder to rest. In the midst of your busy schedule, your body is doing double time, working furiously to physically prepare for the job of nourishing the baby growing in your womb.

In the fast and frenzied pace of this world, allow yourself to submit to the fatigue. Allow it to calm you, settling into the restfulness and peace that come only from God. Thank him for life's slowdowns. †

DAY 57

Popping Buttons

"I eagerly expect and hope that I will in no way be ashamed, but will have sufficient courage so that now as always Christ will be exalted in my body, whether by life or by death."

PHILIPPIANS 1:20

I used to be able to do it, but not today. Despite my nausea and decreased appetite, I had lost the ability to button my pants. Maybe I was just retaining water, or maybe my body was starting to change. Instead of feeling a sense of dread and pulling out my exercise clothes, I was actually thrilled!

Usually, women go to great lengths to hold it all in, trying anything to get zipped up or buttoned together, including jumping up and down or lying down on the bed. But instead, this development had me wanting to share my news with all the world, revealing my bulging, unbuttoned midsection and screaming, "Look, can you see, I can't button!"

Of course, I didn't, realizing that it might appear very odd except, perhaps, to other mothers. Instead, I just wore a loose shirt over my unbuttoned pants or shorts, every so often running my hand over my midsection and smiling at my secret. The button had popped, a sure sign of how God was growing my baby. †

DAY 58

Important Investments

"If you have any encouragement from being united with Christ, if any comfort from his love, if any fellowship with the Spirit, if any tenderness and compassion, then make my joy complete by being like-minded, having the same love, being one in spirit and purpose. Do nothing out of selfish ambition or vain conceit, but in humility consider others better than yourselves."

PHILIPPIANS 2:1–3

If a stranger observed your life, would you easily be recognized as one who lives for Christ rather than one who lives for today? Does the atmosphere you create clearly identify your priorities? Are your fundamental values reconciling with how you budget your time? When it comes down to implementing your beliefs within the routines of your daily life, it's easy to forget what's really important. Do you tend to believe that one day, someday, when you have more time, you'll get to it?

Pregnancy is a great time to realign your life and make changes. Before you bring a baby into your life, take this opportunity to identify and clarify your vision for your life. Look at the way you budget your time and see if it lines up with who you want to be. If you want to spend more time in prayer or reading the Word, do it. If you are tired of trying to keep up with the Joneses, don't. Live your life according to the calling God has put in your heart. †

DAY 59

Demystifying the Myths

"The LORD *is near to all who call on him, to all who call on him in truth."*

PSALM 145:18

You're not even out of the first trimester yet, and already the myths surrounding pregnancy are overwhelming. Does the level of your morning sickness indicate whether you're having a boy or a girl? If you crack open an egg to reveal a double yolk, does it mean that you're having twins? Have you heard the old saying that heartburn is a telltale sign that your baby will have a full head of hair? What is real, what is true?

Listen and enjoy the stories, but always weigh them against the truth of medical knowledge. Some myths are fun but others instill fear, like avoiding baths or raising your hands above your head. Life, too, is full of myths and half truths. When in doubt, we can always check those against the truth in Scripture. God's words are constant and never changing. He is the same yesterday, today, and tomorrow. Your future is in his hands, not the current myth of the day. Look to him for truth. †

High-Definition Living

". . . These are the words of the Amen, the faithful and true witness, the ruler of God's creation. I know your deeds, that you are neither cold nor hot. I wish you were either one or the other! So, because you are lukewarm—neither hot nor cold—I am about to spit you out of my mouth."

REVELATION 3:14–16

Normally I am not a big crier, preferring to remain stoic and strong. But during pregnancy, the tears would drip like a leaky hose. Anything could cause my eyes to water—a touching commercial, a preschooler hugging his mom, a soloist singing in church, or hearing a prayer request.

During pregnancy it seems just about everything is a little more acute—smells, tastes, and emotions. To put it in technology terms, it is almost like going from a regular color TV to a high-definition plasma flat screen. But God has given us all the ability to experience life in high definition all the time; sometimes we just have to try harder to find it.

Mediocrity, dull living, is not what Christ has called us to live. He purposes us to live a passionate, full life, not one spent watching from the sidelines. Pregnancy will be over in a few months, but living a high-definition life doesn't have to end. Live a life of passion, fully engaged in the blessings God has given you to enjoy. †

DAY 61

Faith in Numbers

"For in the gospel a righteousness from God is revealed, a righteousness that is by faith from first to last, just as it is written: 'The righteous will live by faith.'"

ROMANS 1:17

With only three weeks left in the first trimester, you may be anxious to jump ahead, looking forward to the relative security of the next phase of pregnancy, when the risk of miscarriage is decreased. You love this baby so much already, and even though you've been praying throughout your pregnancy, your thoughts may return to fear from time to time. Maybe you try to reassure yourself by looking ahead on the calendar. "If only I get through the weekend, I can stop worrying." Or, "If I just make it to my next doctor's appointment, I'll feel more assured that everything is okay."

Where do you place your faith: in a living God or in a number on a calendar? Which is able to offer you actual security and protection? Of course, it is God. †

DAY 62

Unconditional Love

"The Lord *appeared to us in the past, saying: 'I have loved you with an everlasting love; I have drawn you with loving-kindness.'"*

Jeremiah 31:3

One of the greatest blessings in my life is my grandmother. She was always the one person who made me feel loved, no matter what I had done. When I made mistakes, even something really stupid, she would encourage me to see how I could have made the right choice, and then tell me how talented I was, how proud she was of me, and how much she loved me. Even when she saw me at my worst, she chose to believe the best about me.

She is the same way with all her grandchildren; she chooses to see our potential—what we can be, where we can go—not how we messed up. Because of the way she loved me, I understand more fully the kind of unconditional, unending love God has for us. He loves us exactly where we are today. We don't deserve his love—we've all sinned and fall short. Yet his love is unconditional, ever present, and always available to us. †

DAY 63

Fast Forward

"Do not be anxious about anything, but in everything, by prayer and petition, with thanksgiving, present your requests to God. And the peace of God, which transcends all understanding, will guard your hearts and your minds in Christ Jesus."

PHILIPPIANS 4:6–7

Even though you're only nine weeks pregnant, you've probably been flipping forward in your pregnancy books and are already well versed on what to expect by week twenty-four. Maybe you've even bought some maternity clothes and have them hanging in your closet, ready to wear when you outgrow you regular wardrobe.

Are baby stores like babystyle, Janie and Jack, or Gymboree calling your name? Maybe you've even wandered in to look at the cute infant clothes, eager to own them for your own child, even though you won't need them for many more months. It's understandable—you're excited, you can't wait to experience everything before you. For today, just relax. Put the pregnancy books down. Feel excited expectation, but not anxious expectation. Enjoy this moment in peace, allowing God's peace to consume you. †

DAY 64

Purple Marker?

"For there is one God and one mediator between God and men, the man Christ Jesus, who gave himself as a ransom for all men—the testimony given in its proper time."

1 TIMOTHY 2:5

I glimpsed myself in the mirror one morning as I was undressing before a shower. For a moment, I thought I had purple marker colored on my chest. I rubbed at it and tried to wash it off with soap, but it was still there. Then I leaned in, getting right next to the mirror, and saw that it was my veins, not purple marker. Their increased visibility was the proof that my body was working to meet my baby's needs.

During pregnancy, the blood volume in a woman's body increases between 40 to 50 percent as it supplies nutrients to the baby through the placenta. Your baby depends on your blood during pregnancy, but it is Jesus's blood that ensures a lasting and living hope, the promise of eternal life. His love compelled him to come, live, sacrifice, and die for us, though not a single one of us is worthy. His blood alone was what was required, paying our ransom and rescuing each of us from the grasp of the evil one. Thank you, Jesus, for your precious blood. †

DAY 65

Faith Not Seen

"Now faith is being sure of what we hope for and certain of what we do not see."

HEBREWS 11:1

Do you feel pregnant? Though you can't see the baby, you know he's there. You are confident that a little life is growing and developing deep inside your belly. You have some evidence of that truth. Your own body's physical symptoms such as morning sickness or fatigue promote a feeling of certainty, little reminders that your baby is growing, even though you can't see him with your own eyes. Perhaps you've even been able to detect the sound of a heartbeat with a Doppler monitor.

Isn't that the way God works? Though we can't see him, he is always at work. We can't audibly hear his voice, but we can hear him speaking to us through his Word, the Bible, and we can sense his message for us through the teachings of preachers and teachers. Though he may not physically wrap his arms around us, he blesses us with sisters, friends, and a husband who can. Thank you, God, for even on the days when we don't feel you or see you, you are still there. †

DAY 66

Bouncing Baby

"There are different kinds of gifts, but the same Spirit. There are different kinds of service, but the same LORD. *There are different kinds of working, but the same God works all of them in all men."*

1 CORINTHIANS 12:4–6

Even though you don't feel it, your baby is bouncing and moving around inside your womb. Tiny joints allow her to flex and bend her limbs. Through movement, she is learning what her body can do, learning and exploring within the safety of the protective amniotic sac. Her practice movements help her skeletal and muscular systems develop so that they'll be ready to use once she's born.

God has given you a body equipped for certain unique abilities and talents. Have you fully explored those abilities? Though you know you may have a special gift or talent, are you using it for his glory or shelving it? You've heard the term, "Use it or lose it." This is true for our talents and abilities. We are to constantly train, learn, grow, and practice in order to develop and sharpen the skills God has given us. †

DAY 67

Singing in the Streets

"May my lips overflow with praise, for you teach me your decrees."

PSALM 119:171

I admit it. Instead of a shower singer, I'm a car praiser. Though I may look like a crazed lunatic to other drivers, I just love belting out "LORD, we lift your name on high. . ." while I'm waiting at a stop-light or cruising down the interstate. When my lips are praising him, my focus shifts, releasing whatever daily fire I'm fighting, whatever worry plagues my mind, or any hurt feelings that are stewing.

When my mouth sings of who he is and what he's done for me, I feel like I'm experiencing a little piece of heaven. James 5:13 asks, "Is anyone happy? Let him sing songs of praise." Share your joy about this pregnancy by praising his name today, wherever you are. Let loose in the acoustics of your shower or tune your car radio to a Christian praise station. Praising him in pregnancy is a great way to acclimate the baby to an environment of praise. †

DAY 68

Lifelong Love Affair

"How great is the love the Father has lavished on us, that we should be called children of God! And that is what we are! . . ."

1 JOHN 3:1

This pregnancy is just the beginning of a lifetime love affair. Like all love affairs, there is the instant in-loveness, the giddy, happy, silly feelings. As your child grows and develops, the newness wears off but the in-loveness is still there, growing ever stronger, with fuller knowledge and deeper appreciation of what a unique creation your child is. God makes everyone a unique individual, even identical twins.

This love affair will continue when the child changes from "Mom, you know everything" to "Mom, what do you know?" and will eventually come full circle back to "Mom, what would I do without you?" Through each season and stage, victory and defeat, this child will have you by his side. Whether he's age two, twelve, or thirty-two, you'll be the one who will still be able to wipe a tear and hug the hurt.

God loves you like that. He is your Father, the one who calms your cries, who hears and answers your prayers. You are a child of the Most High God. †

DAY 69

Thinking Thoughts

"Finally, brothers, whatever is true, whatever is noble, whatever is right, whatever is pure, whatever is lovely, whatever is admirable—if anything is excellent or praiseworthy—think about such things."

PHILIPPIANS 4:8

You have thirty weeks to go until the finish line; it may seem like an eternity between here and there. Your maternity clothes have not been bought, or at least worn, yet. At the same time, you can hardly remember what it was like before, to not be pregnant.

The passage of time is such an abstract thing. Have you ever been so focused on a task that an hour passed by before you even realized it? But then there are other times and other activities where the minutes tick by so slowly, the clock seems stuck.

During these weeks of waiting, what would God have you focus your thoughts on? Over the course of the next thirty weeks, you can find joy in the journey, or you can make it a long, weary walk. It's the same amount of time either way, but it's your mind-set that makes the difference. What will you dwell on? The Bible gives you a clear description in Philippians 4:8. †

DAY 70

Hearing the Heartbeat

"I pray that out of his glorious riches he may strengthen you with power through his Spirit in your inner being, so that Christ may dwell in your hearts through faith. And I pray that you, being rooted and established in love, may have power, together with all the saints, to grasp how wide and long and high and deep is the love of Christ."

EPHESIANS 3:16–18

If you were to listen to your stomach with a Doppler instrument this week, you might be able to hear something interesting. Two heartbeats would be audible: your own rhythmic beat and the baby's faster rate. The sound of two heartbeats in one body, beating together, gives such a sense of assurance, such a surge of pride and joy all at once. The heart has always been a symbol of love, and the sound of its life-sustaining energy at work is the sound of pure joy for a mother-to-be.

When Christ is in our hearts, it is the same sense of pride and joy: God in you, in your body, your heart keeping time with his. He works through you, his vessel, to reveal his love, his glory to others. †

DAY 71

Sibling Rivalry

"Keep your lives free from the love of money and be content with what you have, because God has said, 'Never will I leave you; never will I forsake you.'"

Hebrews 13:5

Have you ever listened to the clamor of siblings? "It's not fair!" . . . "I had it first!" . . . "She hit me!" . . . "IT'S MY TURN!" It's enough to make a parent want to pull out her hair.

Aren't we just the same way though? How often are our cries similar in what we say to God? "God, it's not fair. Why did you answer their prayer, but not ours?" Or, "God, I've been faithful, making the right choices, why am I going through this trial?"

Just as you parent each child uniquely according to their God-designed emotional and physical needs, so God parents you. It's hard to be content, to see the blessings you have, when your eyes are focused on what everyone else has, or how their needs have been met. God wants your focus to be on what he has done for you, how he has blessed you, how he has answered your prayers. Instead of clamoring for what is fair, ask God what he wants for your life. †

DAY 72

Medium Fries

"But the fruit of the Spirit is love, joy, peace, patience, kindness, goodness, faithfulness, gentleness and self-control. Against such things there is no law."

GALATIANS 5:22–23

It's generally recommended that moms consume an additional 300 to 500 calories per day during pregnancy. It's kind of like a calorie allowance, an extra amount that you can spend on your daily delicacies. But depending on how you spend it, it doesn't really amount to that much more. One medium order of French fries contains the extra allowance in just one serving. Yikes! You would hardly consider that the nutritional supplement your baby deserves. You get a lot more bang for your buck if you make wise choices. A cup of apple slices has only 110 calories, plus a healthy dose of vitamins and fiber.

Spiritually, how have you been spending your allowance? With twenty-four hours in each day, how much time do you give to God? Have you been saving it all for a super-sized sermon on Sunday? Overdoing it on one day and then fasting the rest of the week? Or are you trying to have a spiritually balanced life, combining prayer, church, the Bible, service, and fellowship? Make good choices for your body and spirit. †

DAY 73

Hunger Pangs

"Blessed are those who hunger and thirst for righteousness, for they will be filled."

MATTHEW 5:6

There's no telling when it will happen, but all of a sudden it returns. You feel hungry, really, really hungry. Maybe it's the smell of juicy steaks on an outdoor grill, or the aroma of freshly baked bread floating out of the bakery, but one day you go from feeling sick and queasy to ravenously desiring food again.

When we make the step of faith to believe in Jesus, a similarly radical change occurs within us, too. We were dead, and through him, we became alive. We moved from darkness into light. We become hungry—ravenous—for his truths, his words, his directions. As we allow him to transform us, it is evident in the way we live our lives.

Have you been hungry for him lately? When was the last time you couldn't wait to dig into the Word or pray, catching up with him? Hunger and thirst for his food. ✝

DAY 74

The Weight of Words

"Reckless words pierce like a sword, but the tongue of the wise brings healing."

PROVERBS 12:18

Do you find yourself carrying on a conversation with the baby in your womb? Throughout his or her life, you will say many, many things. I hope that my children will look back upon the words I've said to them, and I hope they will find them to be a gentle salve, a balm when they are wounded.

I want to make deposits in the bank of good memories, not ones that are memorialized in the "What Mom Did Wrong Hall of Fame." You know, those stories that always start off "Remember when you . . ." Although you may not remember the event at all, the person not only remembers but can tell you exactly what you had for lunch that day and what shirt you were wearing.

Our words are so powerful. It takes only a few thoughtless words to create a lasting, perhaps permanent impression, and many more good words to undo their damage. In a cluster of five or six words, we can encourage or destroy. What will your words be to this child? †

DAY 75

Seasons of Change

"'Your mother was like a vine in your vineyard planted by the water; it was fruitful and full of branches because of abundant water.'"

EZEKIEL 19:10

Growing up, we had a large peach tree in our yard. Some years the tree's branches were heavy, almost touching the ground because they were so full of fruit. Other years, when there had been a drought or a harsh winter, the fruit was small and sparse.

As believers in Christ, we all bear fruit. Some springs are better than others, when we are rich in faith or when we've seen God move in our midst. Other years, we feel like we've been through a dry, cold winter and the fruit we bear is small. Yet, eventually the rain does come and a fruitful season comes again.

What kind of season are you in right now? Do you feel like you are in the spring, fresh and full of him living in you, or perhaps in autumn, full of change, ending one chapter and moving to another? If you are feeling discouraged or tired, as though it's been a long, harsh winter, remember the life growing within you as evidence of the spring to come. †

DAY 76

Taking Notes

"This is what the LORD*, the God of Israel, says: 'Write in a book all the words I have spoken to you.'"*

JEREMIAH 30:2

One of the essential items in my purse is a notepad. It's small, spiral bound, and flips open for easy access. I also keep at least two pencils handy, because whenever I take one out it never seems to make it back in. I use the notebook nearly every day.

During pregnancy, I would write down questions that would pop into my mind, so I didn't forget them during a doctor's visit. Or, if I was feeling queasy, I would record what I had eaten to see if there was a correlation. I would also use it to jot down special Scriptures that seemed to have been penned just for me. When I came across them again later on, it was as though it was a little love note from God to me.

Are you keeping a journal of your pregnancy experience? Be sure to record your prayers for this child. How exciting it will be to return to your journal as your child grows up, and witness God at work. †

DAY 77

Out of the Loop

"Love is patient, love is kind. It does not envy, it does not boast, it is not proud. It is not rude, it is not self-seeking, it is not easily angered, it keeps no record of wrongs."

1 CORINTHIANS 13:4–5

Does your husband feel out of the loop? Everybody is talking about you and the baby, but Dad isn't necessarily the center of interest. He bears the brunt of mood swings, lives with the morning sickness madness, but can't complain because it isn't his body that is going through it. He can't yet place his hand on your tummy to feel the baby move, and there isn't much he can do to ease your discomfort. So how can Dad get back in the loop?

Try to include him in visits with your doctor or midwife, scheduling appointments that meet his schedule. Let Dad find and listen to the baby's heartbeat, giving him a connection to the baby you both created. Encourage him in all his efforts to be a part of this pregnancy. †

DAY 78

Constant Craving

"O God, you are my God, earnestly I seek you; my soul thirsts for you, my body longs for you, in a dry and weary land where there is no water."

PSALM 63:1

Have you found yourself having a taste for unusual foods since you've been pregnant? I constantly crave Mexican food—all the time, not just during pregnancy! I can't help it; it is what happens when you are born and raised in Texas. God just instills that hunger for guacamole, sour cream enchiladas, carne asada, and chips and salsa into your genes. I could literally eat Mexican food every day and still want it the next.

God has also put an unquenchable thirst and hunger for him into our spirits. As God's children we were created to be in a relationship with him. In the beginning Adam and Eve shared a personal, one-on-one relationship with the living God. They saw his face, heard his footsteps, walked and talked with the Most High. The desire to have this kind of intimacy still lives in each of us. We are to constantly crave him. †

DAY 79

Ready to Exhale

"Give ear to my words, O LORD*, consider my sighing. Listen to my cry for help, my King and my God, for to you I pray."*

PSALM 5:1–2

Do you feel a deep breath within you? Do you want to let it out, exhaling deeply, but you can't just yet? You may feel ready to move out of the first trimester with its uncertainty and queasiness, and into the relative security of the second trimester. You're ready to tell the world your news, shouting it from the mountaintops, and move closer to welcoming this baby.

The Word tells us to praise God at all times (Psalm 34:1), to feel like shouting in the moments of gladness, telling all he has done, and to maintain an attitude of praise in the moments of grief when he walks beside us. Right now, you are in a moment of gladness. Praise him! Tell him how thankful you are for placing you in this moment in time. He's brought you to this point and will continue to be with you every week of this pregnancy. †

DAY 80

The New Normal

"Do not lie to each other, since you have taken off your old self with its practices and have put on the new self, which is being renewed in knowledge in the image of its Creator."

COLOSSIANS 3:9–10

Little by little, the "old you" is starting to come back, the you that felt normal. Instead of a roller coaster, with diving drops and racing mountains, you are moving now into a Ferris wheel, where you release the white-knuckle grip and relax. Doesn't it feel good to return to normal, where you can eat easily and stay up late enough to watch American Idol? Isn't it nice to be the person you remember, whose words you recognize and who feels like herself again?

Yet some things are still different. Your body is starting to change shape. Your skin and hair might have a different texture or appearance. These external signs of pregnancy remind you that though you are still the same, you are transforming into a new role. You will always be your own self, but now you will also be a mother.

We also become a new person in Christ. We "look" different—not physically, but in our attitudes and beliefs. We're the same person, but we take on a new role as a child of God. †

DAY 81

3.5 Inches

"From the east I summon a bird of prey; from a far-off land, a man to fulfill my purpose. What I have said, that will I bring about; what I have planned, that will I do."

Isaiah 46:11

Right now, your baby is about the size of your middle finger. Within those few inches, a brain is forming and fingers are growing. It's so much fun to imagine how much bigger your baby will be by this time next week, or by next month, or how in a year you'll be holding her. From those tiny inches of tissue will come a life that glorifies God. While the moments may drag, the years will pass in a blink of an eye, and soon enough she'll be a toddler and then a teen.

Pray today for your baby's development; pray specifically about every aspect of development—physical, emotional, and spiritual. Pray that he or she would grow each day according to God's design and plan, and that you, as this child's parent, would raise a child to fulfill his purpose. †

DAY 82

Shopping Spree

"And my God will meet all your needs according to his glorious riches in Christ Jesus."

PHILIPPIANS 4:19

When I became pregnant the first time, I often found myself roaming the pregnancy and baby aisles of stores. I loved looking at strollers, seeing what kinds of cribs were available, pricing car seats (and everything else!), and making wish lists of what we would need to buy or borrow.

The costs of bringing a baby into the world can be overwhelming. Even after the medical bills for prenatal care and delivery, infants need diapers, clothes, bedding, and car seats, not to mention formula, child care, and equipment. If not sufficiently prepared, the financial future can seem ominous and bewildering.

As you peruse the aisles and catalogs for baby stuff, remember that your provider is not found in the big brick-and-mortar stores or on the Internet. Your provider is the Most High, who is fully able to meet every need. Pray earnestly about your financial situation, and seek his guidance over your spending. †

DAY 83

Daily Buildup

"This righteousness from God comes through faith in Jesus Christ to all who believe. There is no difference, for all have sinned and fall short of the glory of God, and are justified freely by his grace through the redemption that came by Christ Jesus."

ROMANS 3:22–24

As my ten-year-old son cleaned his glasses, he remarked on the buildup of dirt and water spots on the lenses. "Mom," he said, "sin is kind of like the dirt on these glasses. It builds up on your heart and you don't even know it's there until you take the time to look at it."

He was absolutely right. Sometimes we need a fresh perspective in order to see our life clearly, the way that God sees it. We get so used to the way we've been living, that we don't question if it could be different or wrong. How often do we let "little" sins into our life—worry, white lies, greed, envy, strife? Unless we take the time to regularly examine our hearts, asking God to reveal to us what he would have us fix, the sin can build up.

Let pregnancy be your "lens cleaning," the fresh perspective you need to see your life clearly. Ask God to show you the buildup of sin in your life, and address those issues now so that you'll be ready to parent your new child with a clean heart. †

DAY 84

Short-Order Cook

"This, then, is how you should pray: 'Our Father in heaven, hallowed be your name, your kingdom come, your will be done on earth as it is in heaven. Give us today our daily bread. Forgive us our debts, as we also have forgiven our debtors. And lead us not into temptation, but deliver us from the evil one.' For if you forgive men when they sin against you, your heavenly Father will also forgive you. But if you do not forgive men their sins, your Father will not forgive your sins."

MATTHEW 6:9–15

Sometimes it's easy to treat God like a short-order cook. Instead of thanking and praising him, we blurt out requests just like a waitress turning in an order: "Hey, God, I need one order of a healthy baby. I need a side of *extra* energy, and I don't want to be sick anymore. I also need a huge helping of extra income, God, because I don't know how we can afford this child. Oh, and one more thing, I don't want to spend all my time working out after the baby comes, so please, God, I want to gain just twenty-five pounds. Thanks for taking my order, God."

God gave us a manual on how to pray. We are to edify his name; to acknowledge that it is his will we want, not our own; to recognize that he is our provider and fully able to meet our needs. We are to ask for his protection from evil. We are to remember to search our hearts for sin and ask for forgiveness and extend forgiveness. What do your prayers look like? †

SECOND TRIMESTER

Divine Developments

Introduction to the Second Trimester

The second trimester, the interlude between the queasy uncertainty of the beginning of pregnancy and the expansive discomfort of the conclusion, is a time of physical relief for Mom and of rapid growth for Baby. With most of his major organs in place, the second trimester is a time for Baby to practice the skills he'll need to survive outside the womb.

Pregnancy finally feels real, as you begin to look as pregnant as you feel. You'll find these months the ideal time to do most of your active preparation for a new addition to your family, such as shopping for baby items, researching child care options, and decorating a nursery. The most comfortable and energetic period of pregnancy, God probably created this "honeymoon phase" to allow women an opportunity to plan and prepare for their child's arrival before their body becomes physically cumbersome.

Your body's changes reflect the busy activity inside. There's a rapid increase in Baby's size during the second trimester as she more than triples in length, from about 4 inches to nearly 14 inches. Her body straightens out from the curved tadpole of the early weeks into a more recognizable human form; her head and limbs grow more proportionately sized to her torso.

Baby's skin starts the second trimester with a thin, translucent quality, the veins and blood vessels clearly visible. As the weeks pass, the skin thickens and reddens; God protects the tender fetal skin against the watery environment of the womb with two important substances. Lanugo, a fine, downy layer of hair that serves as insulation, will disappear in the third trimester, while vernix, a creamy white substance, coats the skin to provide further protection.

One of the most exquisite moments of pregnancy is the fluttery feeling of movement deep inside your womb. This sensation, called "quickening," confirms the presence of the life growing inside. During the second trimester, you'll feel these bubbles of movement as your baby dances within the watery environment of the amniotic sac, gracefully stretching and stirring her limbs. As her muscles mature, the reflexive action becomes more spontaneous and she'll settle into a regular pattern of rest and activity, often coinciding (or contrasting!) with your daily routine.

Among her daily activities are practice sessions of the skills she'll utilize after birth, such as sucking and swallowing. Her intake of amniotic fluid allows her digestive system and kidneys to begin rudimentary functioning such as producing urine and meconium, the tarry substance that will be excreted in baby's first bowel movement.

DAY 85

A New Chapter

"And you, my son Solomon, acknowledge the God of your father, and serve him with wholehearted devotion and with a willing mind, for the LORD *searches every heart and understands every motive behind the thoughts. If you seek him, he will be found by you; but if you forsake him, he will reject you forever."*

1 CHRONICLES 28:9

The thirteenth week marks the beginning of a new chapter. While you're nowhere near the end of your pregnancy, you're no longer at the beginning as you enter the second trimester. Smack in the middle of pregnancy is such a nice place. You can put the sickness and fatigue behind you and still be comfortable and capable of most activities. Where are you in your spiritual journey? Have you just opened your eyes to God's work in your life? Is he revealing each day how he has loved you from the beginning? Or perhaps you've been walking hand in hand with him for a while. No matter how fresh in faith or deeply established in your relationship with God, his mercies are new every morning.

We don't earn a pedigree in faith based on how long we've believed or how much we've done for Christ. Each day he gives us something new, something fresh, opening our eyes and transforming us ever closer to his image. Every day we can grasp his goodness and get another glimmer of his grace. †

DAY 86

A Song of Praise

"The LORD *is my strength and my song; he has become my salvation. He is my God, and I will praise him, my father's God, and I will exalt him."*

EXODUS 15:2

Growing up under the wing of a musician grandmother instilled a love of music that I want to pass on to my children. During pregnancy, I would often sit with a CD turned up loudly. I'd close my eyes and rest my hands on my belly—the closest I could get to touching my child. Just a few inches separated my world from the baby, safely confined inside my womb. Whether or not the music penetrated to her ears or touched her spirit, it certainly did mine. The calming effects of Bach, or hearing George Winston work his magic on the piano keys, mixed with the sweet tranquility of knowing my child was so close, so safe put me in a frame of mind to really praise God.

In the hecticness of life, praise doesn't simply fall off your tongue. Create moments where your focus is firmly fixed on the blessing. Be where God has placed you right now. What else can you do but praise him? †

DAY 87

Pregnant Pauses

"Find rest, O my soul, in God alone; my hope comes from him."
PSALM 62:5

At what other time in life do you hear people saying, "Slow down," "You need a nap," or "I think you should eat more"? How often are you encouraged to really pamper yourself? Normally our culture propels us to work harder, sleep less, be more efficient. Right now your "job" is to nurture your baby and that literally means slowing down the hectic pace and nurturing yourself. So, sometimes in that quest to do the best job you possibly can in relaxing, slowing down, and growing this baby, it might mean you pamper yourself with a pregnancy massage or an afternoon pedicure.

Those little breaths of air, little pick-me-ups, are actually good for your physical and emotional well-being. Isn't it nice that unlike Mary, Elizabeth, Hannah, or other mothers in the Bible, when you want a minute to pamper yourself, you can go to a nail salon, spa, or even a bookstore for a quick break? †

DAY 88

Timing Travel

"Come and see what God has done, how awesome his works in man's behalf!"

PSALM 66:5

Are you considering taking a trip? The second trimester is the optimal time for travel during pregnancy. With the risks of the first trimester safely behind you and labor months away, why not plan a special trip before Baby is born? It's important to carve time out of your lives, time to spend together as a couple. As your baby gets older, it will become harder and harder to find those moments. There is no better prescription for restoring intimacy and reconnecting than a few days away from work, life, and circumstances.

Go to the mountains and view the majesty of God's handiwork, knowing that the same hands that created those mountains are at work inside of you. Or relax at the beach, reading, resting, and remembering why you love this man, the gift of your oneness growing inside, while reflecting on the gift of God's creation for his created. †

DAY 89

Second Chances

"How much more, then, will the blood of Christ, who through the eternal Spirit offered himself unblemished to God, cleanse our consciences from acts that lead to death, so that we may serve the living God!"

HEBREWS 9:14

Sometimes the enemy is really successful in bringing the mistakes of my past into my mind and memory. I shudder when I reflect on the stupid choices I made as a teenager. Although I also made some good choices, I think of how I would do things differently now, given the chance.

Will my own children listen; will they heed my advice? Or will they have to learn through their own decisions and, sometimes, mistakes? God gives us a choice each day. There is no magic time machine, no rewind button to life. But we do have the choice to begin again every day, despite our mistakes. Through Christ, we are made whole, clean, without blemish or flaw. We are sanctified because his blood covers us. Through Christ, God gives us the ultimate do-over. †

DAY 90

An Empty Canvas

"Train a child in the way he should go, and when he is old he will not turn from it."

PROVERBS 22:6

Have you ever been to a craft store and picked up a blank canvas? Just the feel of one compels you to pick it up and contemplate. There are so many options and possibilities for creating: landscape, still life, portrait, or abstract . . . endless combinations of colors, hues, and patterns . . . so many style options, from realistic to modern to impressionist. What you put on the canvas is entirely your choice. But you can put on the canvas only what you are equipped with. You can't paint a stroke without a brush. If you have only one color, there isn't much opportunity for variation or distinction.

This life you are carrying, your child, is a blank canvas. You are the paintbrush giving your child the life experiences, tools, and encouragement to someday stand alone. What will you equip her with and how? Consider your life lived in the context of this masterpiece. What fundamental features will you impart to your child? †

DAY 91

Your Dwelling Place

"'My dwelling place will be with them; I will be their God, and they will be my people.'"

EZEKIEL 37:27

"There's no place like home." The concept of home brings up all sorts of associations: a place of comfort and rest, a source of pride, a reference for family life. When you think of your home, the place where you pass the minutes of your life, what kind of dwelling place is it? Don't think about the physical description: brick or stucco, ranch or colonial, apartment or condo. Rather, consider the atmosphere. Is it a positive environment? Does it feel safe? Is there harmony? Is there encouragement? Or is the complexion of your home tainted by tension or unease?

What kind of dwelling place will your home be for your baby? A new life will be dwelling with you soon. God gives us all a dwelling place in him, a safe refuge. Allow him to be your dwelling place today, and seek his guidance in establishing your physical dwelling. †

DAY 92

I Love You

"But the man who loves God is known by God."

1 CORINTHIANS 8:3

A year from now you'll have a baby who reaches out for you, whose whole face lights up when you walk into the room. His head will turn and his eyes will scan for yours when he hears your voice. Even in the first few months of life, his love for you will be evident. Soon he will learn to crawl and pull himself into your lap; give you openmouthed, slobbery kisses; and nestle in your arms. Your heart will feel so full you think it could possibly burst. As a mother it is all the payment you ever hope to receive.

Isn't that what God wants from us? He doesn't force us to choose him, to accept Christ. He wants us to desire him, to love him the way a child reaches for his parent. He wants us to seek him out, to light up when he speaks to us through his word, to want to spend time with him in church. Have you told God how much you love him lately? †

DAY 93

A Womb Window

"The heavens declare the glory of God; the skies proclaim the work of his hands."

PSALM 19:1

I always wanted a window into my womb. I knew the baby needed a full forty weeks to grow, but I wanted a sneak peek, a preview, so I could see firsthand what was happening. It's just so hard to imagine. This week the eyebrows are forming on your baby, framing his or her little eyes. Wouldn't it be fun to watch that progress?

Though our bodies don't come equipped with windows, ultrasound images are technology's window to the womb, providing awe-inspiring glimpses and images of your baby in real time. Seeing the glimpses of your future child only heightens your anticipation of meeting face-to-face, waiting for the day of his or her birth.

We are also waiting on glory in heaven. Just as you can't fathom the true joy you'll feel when you hold your child, we cannot begin to fathom the glory that awaits us. Through God's Word, his creation on earth, and the Holy Spirit, little glimpses of his glory are revealed to us each day. †

DAY 94

Stepping-Stones

"So this is what the Sovereign Lord *says: 'See, I lay a stone in Zion, a tested stone, a precious cornerstone for a sure foundation; the one who trusts will never be dismayed.'"*

Isaiah 28:16

As each day of your pregnancy passes, you come a step closer to the final destination: the birth of your child and the beginning of a new life. You can't skip ahead; each day has its own value, an integral piece of the process of growing and developing that is necessary to produce a human being.

You can't have tomorrow without first living through today. Just as each day is built upon the day before it, so it is with our relationship with Christ. He is our cornerstone, the foundation that we build upon. Each day that we grow and develop in our relationship with him brings us one step closer to our own, eternal, new life. †

DAY 95

Make Mamma Happy

"But may the righteous be glad and rejoice before God; may they be happy and joyful."

PSALM 68:3

You've probably heard the saying, "If Mama's not happy, nobody is happy." The reason why there is so much truth in that statement is because Mom is the central element in the home. If Mom is in a bad mood, it throws everybody off. If Mom is sad, she isn't able to play, communicate, and live life as she would otherwise.

There are bound to be times when you feel down, depressed, cross, irritable, or apathetic. Nevertheless, as mother of your household, you will set the tone and the mood for the day. While you can't make your children happy every moment of every day, you can provide an atmosphere conducive to joy. Pray that you would find joy and happiness in the days ahead, that your home would be characterized by contentment and peace, even on the days when the silver lining in the clouds is hard to see. †

DAY 96

Willing Spirit

"Restore to me the joy of your salvation and grant me a willing spirit, to sustain me."

PSALM 51:12

Some days I felt like I was in a really pregnant mood. I was so happy to be pregnant, proudly wearing maternity clothes, talking about pregnancy with other women. Then there were the days when I just wasn't in the mood. I wanted to eat whatever I wanted, forget about choking down my prenatal vitamin, and stop running to the bathroom every twenty minutes. On those days the last thing I wanted to hear was a perfect stranger's horror story of a twenty-four-hour labor gone awry. Regardless of my mood, my body kept on doing the work of growing my baby, continuing to incubate and nourish my child even when my spirit was less than compliant.

Sometimes spiritually we feel the same way; we just don't "feel like it." We're bored or tired or busy. God knows that, and that is why he tells us to pray for a spirit that is willing, to restore our communion with him. He'll continue to grow and nurture us, and wait for our spirit to catch up. †

DAY 97

Drink Up!

"My soul thirsts for God, for the living God. When can I go and meet with God?"

PSALM 42:2

Feeling thirsty? Fluid intake is important during pregnancy. Everything you drink helps support your expanded blood supply, transporting nutrients to your baby. It also ensures that your organs function properly, enabling your kidneys and gastrointestinal system to handle the demands of pregnancy.

Within your womb, your baby thrives in the fluid environment of the amniotic sac. This liquid safety cushion provides not only a safe environment, but ample room for baby to grow. The health of baby is dependent upon good fluid intake.

Just as you and your baby need fluids, your spirit also requires careful hydration. Do you need an extra measure of comfort or a big glass of patience? Just as you supply your baby's need for fluid, so does God supply your spiritual needs. Ask God for what you need today. †

DAY 98

Pregnancy-Induced Amnesia

"So I will always remind you of these things, even though you know them and are firmly established in the truth you now have. I think it is right to refresh your memory as long as I live in the tent of this body, because I know that I will soon put it aside, as our LORD *Jesus Christ has made clear to me."*

2 PETER 1:12–14

Have you noticed that your memory may not be as clear as normal? Have you set your keys down, only to turn around and completely forget where you left them? Or, perhaps found yourself driving along a road, totally unsure of where you are supposed to be going? For me, pregnancy was the beginning of my mommy amnesia. Despite the fact that my calendar is not only on my computer, but also cross-synched on my phone, with constant alarms reminding me of when and where I am supposed to be, I am still hopelessly scattered.

If you've found that you're experiencing some of these mild memory losses, don't panic; it happens to most women. But do you ever find yourself spiritually scattered, forgetting what God has done or what his promises to you are? Sometimes you need to remind yourself, digging into Scripture, and remember that Christ came so that you might have new life. Pause in remembrance of what he has done for you today. †

DAY 99

Skinny Mini

"But the LORD *said to Samuel, 'Do not consider his appearance or his height, for I have rejected him. The* LORD *does not look at the things man looks at. Man looks at the outward appearance, but the* LORD *looks at the heart.'"*

1 SAMUEL 16:7

It's rare to actually feel skinny during a pregnancy; rather, your clothes probably feel fairly tight right now. Buttons are left undone, zippers remain halfway open. Now is the time most women are really starting to accumulate and wear maternity clothing.

The first time you put on maternity clothes, it is such a liberating feeling. You look in the mirror and see these clothes completely swallowing you. You think, "There is *no way* I'll ever actually fit into these clothes!" Enjoy this time to feel like a skinny mini, to be able to enjoy your body, active and fully mobile.

This is a great time during pregnancy to prepare for the days ahead, when you will be more tired and fatigued and walking around won't be as easy as it is now. Isn't it nice to know that God loves you the same now, when you are relatively "skinny," when you are in your fortieth week, feeling large and anything but? God doesn't look at your appearance; he sees only your heart. †

DAY 100

Boxes of Blessings

". . . because of your father's God, who helps you, because of the Almighty, who blesses you with blessings of the heavens above, blessings of the deep that lies below, blessings of the breast and womb."

GENESIS 49:25

Our garage resembled a distribution warehouse for Pampers, with cases of diapers from newborn through size three. No, we didn't win a contest; the inventory was the result of the generosity of those who attended a "diaper shower" for my twin boys. The event provided a dual blessing, saving us money and helping us avoid emergency diaper dashes.

God's blessings come in all shapes and sizes, as subtle as a spectacular sunset or a more tangible reward like a promotion at work. For us, blessings came in cardboard boxes filled with diapers. Regardless of the size, shape, and form of the blessing, we should feel compelled to tell him how grateful we are for the gifts he has given us.

Life has a way of keeping us so busy and distracted that many blessings pass by completely unnoticed. How often has a beautiful spring day passed while you were busy indoors? Has a stack of bills ever tarnished the joy of a pay raise? Be aware of both the little and big blessings in your life today, remembering to thank God for every one. †

DAY 101

Potential Purpose

"And now the LORD *says—he who formed me in the womb to be his servant to bring Jacob back to him and gather Israel to himself, for I am honored in the eyes of the* LORD *and my God has been my strength—"*

ISAIAH 49:5

It's exciting to think of all the possibilities your child has before her. What will she be when she grows up? Perhaps she could be president, an astronaut, a judge, an artist, a doctor, or a teacher. What will she do with her life? Her whole life is before her. The potential for greatness is exciting, isn't it?

As a mom, you want your child to grow into all of her potential, not letting mistakes or missed opportunities impair her abilities. Your child is being created and gifted with talents, abilities, and strengths that will be uniquely hers. As a mom, you have the capacity to help her grow into the person God purposes her to be. Just as your child is formed with a purpose, so are you. God has purposed you for motherhood. God has purposed you for this moment in your life. †

DAY 102

Rubber Bands

"Who is like the wise man? Who knows the explanation of things? Wisdom brightens a man's face and changes its hard appearance."

ECCLESIASTES 8:1

Rubber bands have the most amazing ability to stretch and to contract. They are kind of like a woman's body during pregnancy, slowly expanding out but eventually compressing and returning to a smaller shape. Just like most rubber bands contract, but don't look exactly like they did before use, you will also look a little different after your pregnancy concludes.

Going through any experience changes us, whether it leaves physical or emotional imprints. While your body is physically changing, you are also changing emotionally. Long after this pregnancy has passed, you will never forget the feeling of carrying a child, remembering the way a baby kicks in your womb, or the joy, awe, and wonder of childbirth.

If you allow it, God will work in this experience to change you spiritually, drawing you into a closer relationship with him. Pray that he will stretch you, making you aware of the ways that you need to grow and mature spiritually. †

DAY 103

Nicknames

"For you did not receive a spirit that makes you a slave again to fear, but you received the Spirit of sonship. And by him we cry, 'Abba, Father.' The Spirit himself testifies with our spirit that we are God's children. Now if we are children, then we are heirs—heirs of God and co-heirs with Christ, if indeed we share in his sufferings in order that we may also share in his glory."

ROMANS 8:15–17

Nicknames punctuate many childhood memories. To this day I turn my head when I hear "Suzie Q" in a crowd, even though I know those words aren't meant for me anymore. In utero, our twins were simply Baby A and Baby B. Now our Jon will forever be Jon Jon and James always Jamesie. Though my children may not always enjoy being called by their nicknames, they are all spoken with affection and adoration.

God has words of affection for you, too. He calls you "Mine," "My Child," "Forgiven," "Co-heir of the Kingdom," and more. Relish his adoration and words of affection for you. Seek out these terms of endearment as you're reading the Bible and know that these words of Scripture are meant for you. †

To Test or Not to Test

"For this reason, since the day we heard about you, we have not stopped praying for you and asking God to fill you with the knowledge of his will through all spiritual wisdom and understanding."

COLOSSIANS 1:9

To AFP or not AFP . . . The optional testing of alpha-fetoprotein levels in my blood was a question I debated, deliberated, and considered for many hours. I could see both sides of the issue. On one hand it would be advantageous to know if something was wrong with the baby, so doctors and the medical team could be sufficiently prepared to treat it. But the test was notorious for producing false results. All of the fear and worry would be needless, and ultimately, the results of the test wouldn't change how much I loved and wanted this child.

Are you scared, uncertain, or concerned about the AFP (also called the MSAFP or triple screen) or other medical tests and procedures? Pray that God would give you peace about what the right decision is for you and your family. He has the perfect answer for you. †

Trusting in Technology

"Adam lay with his wife Eve, and she became pregnant and gave birth to Cain. She said, 'With the help of the LORD *I have brought forth a man.'"*

GENESIS 4:1

When I was pregnant I was always so thankful that I wasn't Eve. Who would want to be the first mom? She had no mother or girlfriend to tell her what to expect. She had not a single pregnancy book, Web site, or article to read. Forget sonograms, she didn't even have a doctor to go to for checkups! The one thing she did have was God, and that was enough. Eve, before the Fall, had personally walked and talked with God. She knew fully that he was enough.

Sometimes it is easy to glean our faith from technology. We begin to trust in the sonographer, doctor, and test results more than we trust in God. Where is your trust today? †

DAY 106

Creating Contentment

"Death and Destruction are never satisfied, and neither are the eyes of man."

PROVERBS 27:20

We were not created to be content creatures. Our culture capitalizes on our lust for more. Watch television at any time of the day and there are commercials and infomercials designed to convince us that we can't be beautiful, successful, or happy unless we buy the right floor polish, tooth whitener, or soda. And because all parents want the best for their child, marketers capitalize on their desire by offering designer baby clothes, luxury-model strollers, mahogany nursery furniture and other unnecessary—and expensive—items for babies. It is an appetite that can never be satisfied in the flesh.

In Christ we are liberated from the quest for more. In Christ, we have enough, we are satisfied. In Christ, our eyes are fixed on him, not on what we do not have. Have your eyes slowly been shifting off of him, to the circumstances or things of this world? Recast your eyes and find his face. Fix your eyes on the Eternal. †

Daily Do-Overs

"All a man's ways seem right to him, but the Lord *weighs the heart."*

Proverbs 21:2

There are no do-overs for the big mistakes in life, but as a mom you'll have the opportunity for each day to be a clean slate. If on one day you make a mistake, for example, if you're in a bad mood or didn't find the time to interact or bond with your child the way you wished, the next day is another chance.

Everybody has bad days. Everybody makes mistakes, says words she regrets, or behaves badly. What you can do is apologize for the harsh words that were spoken. You can show through your actions of today that you desire to make up for your mistake of yesterday. Focus on your fresh beginning today, not on what you did wrong yesterday. †

DAY 108

Skipping the Story

"The end of a matter is better than its beginning, and patience is better than pride."

ECCLESIASTES 7:8

Now that you've experienced the beginning of your pregnancy and had a taste of the middle trimester, you may feel ready just to jump to the ending. Enough being pregnant, let's move on to being a mom! Just as it would ruin a great novel if you read only the first and last pages, missing the story in between, this part of pregnancy should not be skipped or glossed over either. The end will come soon enough.

Unlike a book, once each day passes, you can't go back and reread a particular section or chapter. Each day of waiting makes the reward of holding your baby that much sweeter. Every kick you feel helps you bond with your baby before she ever touches your arms. Each glimpse of the sonogram helps your eyes see what your arms long to feel. You get one chance to experience each day. Enjoy this time, the story of your body's physical and mental preparation for parenting. †

Insurance Policies

"He who overcomes will, like them, be dressed in white. I will never blot out his name from the book of life, but will acknowledge his name before my Father and his angels."

REVELATION 3:5

Now that your family is growing, it is time to think about the practical matters in life. Do you need a new car? You've realized that the two-seater sports coupe won't accommodate a new car seat. What about life insurance? All parents owe their children the gift of financial security. Have you written a will? Make it a point to have an open discussion with your husband about your own care, should you become terminally ill. Who will care for your children in case both of you are involved in a tragedy? How will your assets be handled? Preparing for the future, planning security for your family, demonstrates your love for them.

Christ, too, has planned for us. He loves us so much that he has prepared a place for us. Through him we have a future, an insurance policy for eternal life. When you choose Christ, your name is written into the book of life; you are his. †

DAY 110

Little Surprises

"Therefore, as God's chosen people, holy and dearly loved, clothe yourselves with compassion, kindness, humility, gentleness and patience."

COLOSSIANS 3:12

One hot summer day, our family was vacationing in the mountains. When my husband was called away on business, I was left alone with four kids eager to hit the trails despite a heat wave. After a long day of hiking and caring for four hungry and tired kids, a sick dog and rude residents, I was ready to fly home.

My brother-in-law and his wife stopped by just as I was putting the kids to bed. When I was finished reading to the kids, I came out to the porch to find a plate of cheese, crackers, and fruit and a glass of wine. Such a simple act had never been appreciated more. It's often those simple things that mean the most: a kind word spoken in a moment of deep despair or an extra pair of hands helping with a child when you most need it. These small random acts of kindness make living bearable when you feel ready to give up. In the Bible, we can find those words of encouragement from God, his kind reminders that he loves us and that we need not despair. †

DAY 111

Subtle Signs

"In the same way, let your light shine before men, that they may see your good deeds and praise your Father in heaven."

MATTHEW 5:16

Are you starting to feel a strange sensation, like little bubbles in your belly? At first it is hard to discern if you are feeling the baby or a little leftover from lunch. As your baby grows, it will become easier to determine that it is the baby moving. The little flutters are such a wonderful reassurance of the life growing and thriving within you.

Just as your child is thriving within you, showing signs evidencing her development, you should be growing spiritually too. What signs in your life demonstrate that you are growing spiritually? Perhaps you've found patience in traffic that normally would send you over the edge. Or maybe you've been able to extend forgiveness and grace to someone who has hurt you. Through Christ, we have the amazing ability to thrive and grow, reflecting his light and love in the way that we lead our lives. †

DAY 112

A Direct Line

"Hannah was praying in her heart, and her lips were moving but her voice was not heard."

1 SAMUEL 1:13

In our home we have three cordless telephones, yet every time the phone rings, someone in the house undoubtedly shouts, "Where's the phone?" Somehow they all mysteriously vanish into the far recesses, beneath pillows, in the laundry room, or in a child's closet.

During pregnancy, the phone was practically attached to my ear. I would call my friends at the slightest twinge, saying, "I felt this today, what about you? Have you felt that before?" When I was pregnant with my twins, the phone served as a lifeline to the doctor's office, providing immediate answers to my questions and concerns.

With God, isn't it nice that we don't have to worry about losing our "phone," our connection to communication with him? Our access to him is more direct than calling a friend or a doctor's office. He is always there; all we have to do is call on him. Whether we cry out to him audibly or within our hearts, he always hears what we have to say. †

DAY 113

Baby Fat

"I have hidden your word in my heart that I might not sin against you."

PSALM 119:11

As your baby's body grows, a layer of fat develops under his skin, which serves a very important purpose. It'll provide a layer of insulation and eventually help him regulate and maintain his body temperature.

Have you ever noticed that God's Word, like the layer of baby fat, serves much the same purpose? Hidden in your heart, the words you have poured into your soul serve to insulate and protect you when you are going through a trial or are having a moment of doubt. Those words and passages help us to find comfort in him in our time of need, protecting us and reminding us of his goodness. The words also come to us in times when we may be tempted to sin, reminding us to follow his will in making the right choice.

Have you spent time lately hiding God's Word in your heart? Spend some time building up your storehouses, so that in times of need you will not forget what his promises are for you. †

DAY 114

Sick of Sweat

"But thanks be to God, who always leads us in triumphal procession in Christ and through us spreads everywhere the fragrance of the knowledge of him."

2 CORINTHIANS 2:14

Who knew that pregnancy could make you sweat like a marathon runner when all you did was walk from the mall to your car in the parking lot? During pregnancy it is normal to notice an increased amount of sweat and other bodily secretions. It isn't the nicest part of pregnancy; in fact, it rates right up there with puffy cheeks and swollen ankles. Stinky sweat is not really what you had envisioned when you became pregnant. Women usually like to smell fresh and sweet, not stinky and sweaty.

To the world, Christians are the fragrance of Christ. Everywhere we go, with everyone we encounter, we leave a remnant behind, a scent by which we'll be remembered. As you interact in your friendships, work relationships, even with the gas station attendant, you have a chance to be the fragrance of Christ, a subtle reminder of him. †

Creative Creation

"So God created man in his own image, in the image of God he created him; male and female he created them."

Genesis 1:27

God is so amazing in the way that he attends to even the smallest details of his creation. Moment by moment this child is being created in God's own image. Every detail bringing her closer to the day of birth is continually being perfected and finessed, from tiny fingernails at the tips of her fingers to myelin, a protective barrier forming around her nerves.

Of all the amazing creatures that God created, he made us to be like him. We are not like the birds of the air or the fish of the sea. We are creatures created in his likeness, made to have fellowship and a relationship with him. God did not create us to serve as his pets, but as his companions. †

DAY 116

Perfection Is Not Required

"'I am the LORD*'s servant,' Mary answered. 'May it be to me as you have said.' Then the angel left her."*

LUKE 1:38

Thankfully, perfection is not a requirement on the resume for motherhood. Every woman falls short of the ideal image. None of us comes to the role of motherhood as a perfect role model or with the perfect loving and patient spirit. Fortunately, we can go to God with our imperfections.

He knows what you need more of. He knows where you hurt and how to heal those hurts so that hurtful cycles in your own life are not repeated again in your child's life. He does not require you to be perfect, only willing and ready to love.

God is giving you the charge of his creation, entrusting you with the ability to help grow, nurture, and teach your child. What is required to be a mom? Only that you are willing to give your daily best, desiring to serve God in this most important job as mother. All of us will make mistakes; the important thing is that you pick up and move on. †

Sleeping Soundly

". . . 'Let the beloved of the LORD *rest secure in him, for he shields him all day long, and the one the* LORD *loves rests between his shoulders.'"*

DEUTERONOMY 33:12

During the second trimester, your baby is beginning to develop sleeping patterns. As you begin to feel your baby move more, you will become aware of when she is sleeping and awake, when she is feeling energetic, and when she has the hiccups. Just through feeling your baby move, you will begin to learn so much about her and her personality.

What do your sleeping patterns say about you? Are you fitful and restless, full of worry and stress? When you lie down to sleep, do you toss and turn, unable to find peace because the day's events and life stresses continue to race through your mind? Or when you sleep, is your rest calm because you have trusted in God? If you can't sleep right now due to physical discomfort or stress, pick up his Word and find him. Pray for peace; release to God anything that is disrupting your rest. Sleep soundly in his presence. †

DAY 118

He Is Better

"One thing I ask of the LORD, *this is what I seek: that I may dwell in the house of the* LORD *all the days of my life, to gaze upon the beauty of the* LORD *and to seek him in his temple."*

PSALM 27:4

The world is a tempting place, isn't it? It's hard for me to walk into a supermarket and stick to my grocery list without throwing in additional items that look appealing or are a good bargain. The bigger attractions—like home improvements, the latest fashions, a new car, or vacations—are always readily available for purchase, even from the comfort of a computer. We've unlearned patience. We've forgotten how to save up for big purchases and sacrifice for what we want.

What does your heart desire? Are you seeking God, or are you seeking the world's possessions? Are your eyes fixed upon the cross, or are they gazing upon futile fashions? This week focus on him, allowing the peripheral concerns in your life to decrease. God is better. †

DAY 119

Rattle, Rattle

"As a prisoner for the Lord, *then, I urge you to live a life worthy of the calling you have received. Be completely humble and gentle; be patient, bearing with one another in love. Make every effort to keep the unity of the Spirit through the bond of peace."*

Ephesians 4:1–3

My husband always thought the first rattle he heard would be the baby's toy, not the sound of an antacid bottle. But during my pregnancy, he would wake up several times a night to hear the familiar *rattle, rattle* of the Tums bottle. The pills were an integral part of my pregnancy. Every night, without fail, I would have severe heartburn. A few Tums would always do the trick and I could easily fall back asleep again. It didn't matter what I ate or drank, with each and every pregnancy I always had my Tums nearby to ease the symptoms.

How often do we cause heartache to Christ? Is that burning sensation what he feels when he watches me choose something that is not his way? Do I make his heart hurt? I wonder how it must make him feel when I know the cost of my sin and yet I choose it anyway. Pray today for God to help you walk in a way that does not cause him heartache. †

Under or Over?

"For the kingdom of God is not a matter of eating and drinking, but of righteousness, peace and joy in the Holy Spirit, because anyone who serves Christ in this way is pleasing to God and approved by men."

ROMANS 14:17–18

How much weight have you gained? Your doctor or midwife will advise you whether you are over, under, or right on track in this area. Remember to make good, healthy, nourishing choices each day. Without eating too much extra, you can make every calorie you consume count for the baby.

Just as you should have a balanced diet, are you having a balanced life right now? In addition to eating well, are you remembering to rest, to slow down and allow your body to physically rejuvenate? Are you spending time with your husband, family, and friends? Are you giving back to your community? Most importantly, are you allotting time for your spirit, finding quiet time to spend with God? Try to bring balance into your life today. †

Church Home

"As for Titus, he is my partner and fellow worker among you; as for our brothers, they are representatives of the churches and an honor to Christ. Therefore show these men the proof of your love and the reason for our pride in you, so that the churches can see it."

2 CORINTHIANS 8:23–24

When my husband and I were first married, we joined a Sunday school class for young married couples. It provided a great network of like-minded friends who were newlyweds like us, and also became the framework for the friendships of my life.

We found that two other couples were expecting babies within weeks of our own due date. It was such a joy to have other women to talk to, pray with, and share pregnancy stories with. After our babies were born, we met weekly at each other's houses with our children. Later, during my pregnancy with my twins, these same two ladies rallied around me with support for my family during my hospitalization. Our church family provided meals and, most important of all, prayer, covering the lives of our babies.

Your baby will be born into your genetic family, but what about your church family? Having a church family goes far beyond just someone to say hi to on Sunday, but having an extended network of people—sisters and brothers in Christ—who will shower you with love when you need it the most. †

Dizzy Days

". . . he who made the Pleiades and Orion, who turns blackness into dawn and darkens day into night, who calls for the waters of the sea and pours them out over the face of the land—the LORD *is his name—"*

AMOS 5:8

It is normal to have moments of dizziness and light-headedness during pregnancy, as your hormones change your blood volume and your expanding uterus puts pressure on blood vessels. Often when I stood up, everything would go black and I would have to grab hold of a chair or the wall until things came back into focus. That feeling of encroaching darkness and physical unsteadiness was frightening but always temporary.

Sometimes life is like that—we go through seasons where we have to just hold on, knowing that God has an answer and that soon it will be revealed. Though everything looks dark and we feel completely lost, he is still in control and will bring light to the situation. Look to him to clarify your focus when things feel unbalanced or off-kilter. †

Leaky Glass

"If you obey my commands, you will remain in my love, just as I have obeyed my Father's commands and remain in his love. I have told you this so that my joy may be in you and that your joy may be complete."

JOHN 15:10–11

One of the greatest perks of following Christ is the joy he gives us. It doesn't matter what is going on around us and our family, with Christ we can have joy anytime, in any situation. Yet, sometimes as Christians we give up this perk. We try to glean joy from our circumstances, not from the one who makes our joy complete.

It is kind of like trying to fill a leaky glass with water. No matter how long the faucet is on, the glass will never be full. We need to seal the leaks, remembering that our joy is not dependent upon what we have or what we are going through, but because of what was done for us on the cross.

Being pregnant and becoming a mother may bring you great joy. But by walking in obedience to his commands and living a life for his glory, your joy will be complete. †

DAY 124

Increase Absorption

"Yet a time is coming and has now come when the true worshipers will worship the Father in spirit and truth, for they are the kind of worshipers the Father seeks. God is spirit, and his worshipers must worship in spirit and in truth."

JOHN 4:23–24

Iron intake is an important element of prenatal health, supplying the maternal bloodstream with sufficient stores of oxygen and boosting Baby's birth weight. Vitamin C, found in citrus fruit like oranges and grapefruit, helps increase the absorption of iron whereas dairy products inhibit it, so it's important to take iron supplements with the right combination of food.

Just as you want to ensure that your diet promotes the optimal absorption of the vitamins and minerals your body—and your baby—needs, it's important to have good absorption of the things God puts in your life as well. When you go into the house of God, prepare your spirit for worship so that you can receive the message, praise him as he deserves, and excitedly expect "the Great I Am" to join in the service. If you are frazzled, late, grumpy, worried about your hair or the toddler in child care, you won't be able to easily absorb what God is trying to do for you. Just as vitamin C makes iron supplements more effective, having an appropriately prepared state of mind before a church gathering helps enhance your spiritual experience. †

DAY 125

Daily Arsenal

"Let love and faithfulness never leave you; bind them around your neck, write them on the tablet of your heart."

PROVERBS 3:3

If you are anything like me, your handbag is probably full of all of the things you need for each day. There are the staples—wallet, hairbrush, pen and paper—and then there are those items that you need for the phase of life you are in. In a few months your diaper bag will double as your handbag, housing not only your wallet, but diapers, bottles, pacifiers, and more. While you're pregnant, it can't hurt to carry a water bottle and a few healthy snacks with you. Make your own trail mix with items you like—nuts, raisins, and granola. Or pack a small box or two of nonsugary cereals, which provide a great boost when you need a snack on the go.

Also include spiritual snacks for the moments when you have pangs of worry that something is wrong or when you are in the doctor's office and just need to read a reminder of God's message for you. Download a Bible to your PDA or buy a pocket-sized Bible for easy access to spiritual snacks throughout your day. †

DAY 126

A Safe Ear

"Thus they bring judgment on themselves, because they have broken their first pledge. Besides, they get into the habit of being idle and going about from house to house. And not only do they become idlers, but also gossips and busybodies, saying things they ought not to."

1 TIMOTHY 5:12–13

Women love to talk—about themselves, about pregnancy, about motherhood. But sometimes it's uncomfortable to share your innermost thoughts with others, because of how they react to your words. You may feel judged or defensive, explaining and justifying why you feel a certain way. Isn't it nice that when you go to God, you can pour out every concern regardless of how ridiculous it may sound to someone else? His ear is safe; he doesn't judge and he keeps what you tell him in strict confidence.

He knows your heart and has the perfect antidote to your fear. Sometimes the answer comes in the form of a calming Scripture passage, reassurance from a trusted friend, an answer from the doctor, or simply a sense of peace that only he can give.

Just as we want a safe ear to hear us, sometimes friends and associates, or one day, your child, will seek you out as a listening ear. Ask God to help you in those situations, to keep confidences, to be a safe ear. †

Building Brain and Body

"You will keep in perfect peace him whose mind is steadfast, because he trusts in you."

ISAIAH 26:3

During the summertime I ask my kids to do two important things. First, whether it is through swimming, baseball, or soccer, they need to exercise. Second, they need to keep their brains sharp. I always hear a protesting, "Mommmmmmm, why do we have to do this?" and I'm always ready with the answer: "Because we need to keep your body sharp and fit and your brain sharp and fit. If you don't use it, you lose it."

Though they don't necessarily like having to do "work" in the summertime, it always pays off when school starts back up. As adults, it's a little harder to ensure we do those things on a daily basis, especially during pregnancy, when your mind is so focused on having a baby. Keep your mind sharp by challenging yourself throughout this pregnancy. Ever wanted to learn a language? Why not try now, listening to tapes and practicing out loud in a conversation with your baby? What about music lessons? Pregnancy is a great time to challenge yourself. Expand your focus beyond the pile of pregnancy books. †

DAY 128

Sonogram Staging

"In the morning, O Lord, *you hear my voice; in the morning I lay my requests before you and wait in expectation."*

Psalm 5:3

Right before you crawl aboard a theme-park ride, there is usually a little preride show, often in a dark room, where they try to psyche you up for the thrilling experience ahead. You know that within moments you'll be plunging into the darkened abyss, holding onto the bar for what is sure to be an exciting ride.

Do you feel like that now? For the last five months you've been carrying this child, reading baby books, and wondering if you are having a boy or a girl. Soon you'll most likely have a sonogram, a peek at the child inside. You may discover whether it's a girl or a boy. Are you excited, scared? Is your heart set on a particular gender?

Remind yourself that God, the ultimate Creator, who knows how to knit and form your child, also knows exactly what you need. He knows how to build and complete your family and is giving you exactly what he purposes. Prepare your heart to feel gladness at whatever the news is, rather than what you think you might need. †

Red Flags

"But the Counselor, the Holy Spirit, whom the Father will send in my name, will teach you all things and will remind you of everything I have said to you."

JOHN 14:26

The increased blood production in your body during pregnancy can put pressure and stress on your veins. As a result, varicose veins often manifest themselves during pregnancy. They can be unsightly and painful and are one of the parts of pregnancy that we would rather not experience.

The throbbing and pulsing of the veins you experience when standing or being on your feet too long remind you to give your legs a break. The Holy Spirit works much like that in our life, giving us little red flags in our spirit. When we feel a sense in our spirit that we shouldn't go somewhere or do something, often that is the Holy Spirit's way of prompting us to seek a different outcome.

Just as we can hurt our bodies when we don't listen to the physical cues of overexertion, we are in jeopardy of incurring consequences when we don't listen to the Holy Spirit. Instead of ignoring the warning signs, take a moment to hear what the Holy Spirit is trying to tell you and pray about the direction you should go in. †

DAY 130

Baby's Ears

"But Christ is faithful as a son over God's house. And we are his house, if we hold on to our courage and the hope of which we boast. So, as the Holy Spirit says: 'Today, if you hear his voice, do not harden your hearts. . . .'"

HEBREWS 3:6–8

You might think the womb is a quiet, silent place, but actually there is plenty of sound to be experienced, from the whooshing rhythm of your heartbeat to the gurgles of your digestive system. Over his lifetime, your child's ears will hear many words: words of truth, words of encouragement, words of praise, but also harsh words, lies, and words of evil. His ears will hear your voice and eventually learn to discern not only your voice, but also the voice of right and wrong, the voice from above, and the voice of the world.

God speaks to us through his Word, through people, and through situations. His voice breathes hope, giving life to a future. The world's powerful voice, stemming from the media and our culture, instills hopelessness, disdain, and false truths. As your baby's ears develop, pray that he or she would learn to hear the voice of the LORD, that your child's heart would discern the right way, not the world's way. Pray that your child's ears would be protected. †

Holding Tank

"I have set you an example that you should do as I have done for you. I tell you the truth, no servant is greater than his master, nor is a messenger greater than the one who sent him. Now that you know these things, you will be blessed if you do them."

JOHN 13:15–17

Are you starting to feel like a holding tank? Some days it would be nice if you could just be like a bird taking a break from sitting on the eggs in the nest and get up and move around before going back to the full-time job of growing your baby. Unfortunately, growing a baby is a full-time job, requiring 100 percent of your time and dedication. There is no way to take the night off and eat or drink whatever you would like.

When you are tempted to feel sorry for yourself, remember that it is a privilege to grow this child. Just as Christ came to serve us, not to be served, you have the opportunity to do the same. Though Christ deserved a crown of glory, a throne, and adoration from all life on Earth, instead he washed feet, healed the sick, preached to the masses, gave the bread of life, loved the unlovable, and taught the ugly. Appreciate the privilege of being able to serve by carrying this life. †

DAY 132

Comfort Food

"When anxiety was great within me, your consolation brought joy to my soul."

PSALM 94:19

When I am worried about something or feeling down, I always seem to find myself in front of the pantry doors. I open them up, stand there for about ten minutes, hungry for something. Though I might try to eat comfort food—potato chips or cookies—it isn't what I am really hungering for.

I am hungry for God's peace, to know that regardless of the outcome in any given situation, everything will be okay. Are you in need of God's comfort food right now? With a sonogram and other important assessments of your pregnancy around the corner, you may feel uneasy, longing for the fullness of his peace. In these times, as you encounter worries or uneasiness, remember that God has the comfort you are seeking. †

DAY 133

Preserving the Past

"Remember the days of old; consider the generations long past. Ask your father and he will tell you, your elders, and they will explain to you."

Deuteronomy 32:7

What do you really know about your parents or grandparents? Sure you grew up with them and heard stories of the past, but do you really know who they were? Though I was very close to my grandparents, I always saw them as my grandparents, not as individuals with passions and beliefs. It wasn't until years after my grandfather passed away that I came into possession of his letters to my grandmother during World War II. His written words gave me a snapshot of the past, a picture of who he was, what he believed, what his principles were, and how deeply and passionately he loved my grandmother.

Consider your own journey. You are about to become a mother, and perhaps one day a grandmother. How can you preserve a part of you, a legacy to be shared with your children and grandchildren? Will they know that you loved God? What will be remembered? †

DAY 134

American Idols

"And now, O Israel, what does the LORD *your God ask of you but to fear the* LORD *your God, to walk in all his ways, to love him, to serve the* LORD *your God with all your heart and with all your soul . . ."*

DEUTERONOMY 10:12

God asks one thing of each of us, that we love him with all our heart, soul, and might. We are not supposed to worship other gods or idols. Seems easy enough, right? In this day and age, who would worship statues of stone or cast metal, something created by man's own hands?

Yet, we all have idols, some of which may have begun to slowly creep into your life, incrementally increasing in importance. American idols look different from the idols of yesteryear. If one were to look at American lives and see where the time and attention, assets and resources are allocated, one might surmise that our idols are cars, careers, television, or even sports.

What in your life may have become an idol? How can you balance your life once again, allowing God to be the center, not the idols? †

A Perfect Plumb Line

"And the LORD *asked me, 'What do you see, Amos?' 'A plumb line,' I replied. Then the* LORD *said, 'Look, I am setting a plumb line among my people Israel; I will spare them no longer.'"*

AMOS 7:8

The second trimester is an ideal time to start preparing a nursery for baby. If your decorating plans include painting stripes or hanging wallpaper, you may find a plumb line to be a useful tool. Weighted with a small stone, the force of gravity pulls a string into a perfectly straight vertical. The plumb line is so essential because if you don't have the first line straight, the rest of the lines will be crooked as well. The plumb line serves as a guide for all of the other lines in the room.

In life, we have the perfect plumb line, the standard against which we can measure everything else. Christ is the perfect standard, the unblemished and perfect lamb. He is the one who knows every temptation we ever face, because he faced them too and yet never sinned. Isn't it wonderful to have a perfect plumb line? †

DAY 136

Faithful Fasting

"So we fasted and petitioned our God about this, and he answered our prayer."

EZRA 8:23

I have to admit, fasting is one of the areas in my spiritual life that I have struggled with. When I skip more than one meal, I usually get the shakes and feel lightheaded. What a relief it was during pregnancy to know that, for medical reasons, I could not fast; it was not allowed. Yet, then the LORD brought to my attention other ways of fasting, like withholding a treat, perhaps desserts or a favorite staple on my menu. Fasting didn't even have to be about food. I could fast financially, by not purchasing things I would normally purchase.

Fasting is about giving up something, routinely, sacrificially, while praying for an outcome. The best part about fasting is that each time you refrain from that item, you are reminded of what you are praying for, and inspired to focus on and pray for that request. †

DAY 137

Your Will Be Done

"Samuel told all the words of the LORD *to the people who were asking him for a king."*

1 SAMUEL 8:10

The Israelites begged God for a king when he had already given them a government of judges. Hearing their outcry, God gave them what they wanted, and in the end, they learned that their answer was not as good as God's. Like the Israelites who clamored for a king, sometimes we forget that God's will is better than our own solutions. We look for the quick fix or the easy answer. But there is no shortcut through pregnancy, no fast forward or skip buttons; the moments spent in struggle are producing a worthwhile reward. Unlike pregnancy where there is a definitive end to the waiting, some struggles seem to draw out month after month despite the prayers and the pleading.

Have you been clamoring, begging, pleading with God for something lately? Sometimes his no, as much as we don't want to hear it, is far better than a yes. Though we don't see what he has in store, we do know it is for our good and benefit. Ask him today for his will to be done. †

DAY 138

From the Mouths of Babes

". . . 'I will watch my ways and keep my tongue from sin. . . .'"

PSALM 39:1

While babysitting a baby bird that my brother-in-law was nursing back to health, I complained. I said I didn't like the way the grackle smelled or the mess it made or the way it squawked every few minutes for more food. Furthermore, it was just plain ugly.

My lips were too loose. My six-year-old responded, "Mommy, he can't help it that he is ugly. God just made him that way. It's not his fault." Immediately convicted of my mean-spirited comment, I apologized to the bird and to my son. Just like the grackle, I make messes, I continuously squawk to God, and I always have needs, but I didn't think about that when I allowed ugly words to quickly fall off my tongue.

Conversations have the ability to quickly turn in a direction we don't want them to go. It's easy to allow negativity, criticism, and cutting remarks to flow off our lips, and then spend the rest of the day in regret. What have your conversations been covering lately? What kind of words have you used? Are they pleasing to Christ? †

DAY 139

With All of Me

"Teacher, which is the greatest commandment in the Law?" Jesus replied: "'Love the Lord *your God with all your heart and with all your soul and with all your mind.' This is the first and greatest commandment.'"*

Matthew 22:36–38

With all of my heart . . . I know that is how I am supposed to love God. I don't want to hold anything back; I want him to rule over every area in my life. But sometimes I find myself holding on to a small piece. I give him everything in my life, and yet I refuse to release my grip on a certain area.

Do you ever find yourself doing that? It's like you put God in control over your finances, your marriage, your job, but maybe with this pregnancy, you find that you are still holding on, wanting to control the outcome by your actions.

God instructs us to love him with all of our being. He should be first in our finances, first in our marriage, first in our priorities, first in everything. Is he first right now? Has something come in and rearranged the standings, perhaps shifting pregnancy, marriage, or friendships above him? Take a good look at your life. Have you given him all of your heart? †

DAY 140

Sucking In

"Who of you by worrying can add a single hour to his life?"
LUKE 12:25

I felt like a puffer fish in pregnancy. I'd spend no less than five minutes a day in front of the mirror, sucking in my cheeks. For a brief few minutes I could see the old me, but as soon as I exhaled, those cheeks filled back out. Puffiness was never one of those pregnancy hallmarks I was especially excited about. Yet, it was a side effect of pregnancy, a physical manifestation of what was going on inside of me. Physical signs often reveal what is going on internally. Whenever I am stressed, my hairdresser can look at my hair and know immediately. Or if I'm feeling down, I tend to eat less or eat more.

Do you have any physical symptoms that might be manifestations of emotional conflict? What have you been holding on to instead of releasing to God? Perhaps you have harbored concern over Baby, finances, or work? Look at your life and see if there are things going on that you don't even recognize and prayerfully give them to God. You'll feel better for it. †

DAY 141

Is That My Mother?

"For God did not give us a spirit of timidity, but a spirit of power, of love and of self-discipline."

2 TIMOTHY 1:7

Do you ever catch a glimpse of yourself in the mirror and do a double take when the reflection looking back at you has a striking resemblance to your mother? Perhaps it is the way your shoulders are shaped, or your cheekbones, or the way your hips are set . . . just something distinctive about your mom that you now see in yourself. Though you may not recognize the nonphysical traits as easily, you also resemble her in other areas, perhaps your sense of humor or her gentle spirit.

During these days of pregnancy, think about those traits you want your children to adopt in their own hearts. What distinguishing characteristics can you help imprint and form in their character? Through Christ, you have been given a spirit of power, love, and self-discipline. These traits are not always typical of human nature, but because of Christ, they now define you. You have the ability to teach this child about Christ, allowing him or her to receive the greatest gift of all, an eternal imprint. †

DAY 142

Painful Reminders

"He rescued me from my powerful enemy, from my foes, who were too strong for me. They confronted me in the day of my disaster, but the LORD *was my support."*

2 SAMUEL 22:18–19

Can pain be good? For instance, if your hand is touching a hot stovetop, your nerve endings alert you to remove your hand. Or if you are exercising too strenuously the continuous and sudden Braxton Hicks contractions compel you to stop or slow down. Sometimes pain happens and it prompts another reaction: it drives you to rely on God.

We are a blessed people, who live in a blessed society. For many people, the more blessings they receive, the less they see a need for God in their lives. When pain happens, whether in the form of the death of a loved one, a job loss, a betrayal, or a disappointment, the pain is a reminder to turn to him, the only true source of peace and comfort. Though you may be excited about your pregnancy, perhaps a struggle in your marriage, finances, or work issues have stolen the blessing of your pregnancy. Lean on God during these problems, the One who is strong enough to support you through the darkest trial. †

A Due Reward

"Rejoice and be glad, because great is your reward in heaven, for in the same way they persecuted the prophets who were before you."
MATTHEW 5:12

The rewards of pregnancy are pretty clear; at the end of nine months, you'll hold a son or a daughter in your arms. But many times in life, rewards don't always seem so clearly divided into neat "give and get" categories. Doesn't it seem like some people get away with murder? You may feel like you're running the race, making the right choices, yet despite all of your hard work and right choices, you can't seem to come out ahead. Yet every day you see other people flourishing, even those lacking integrity and values, or even despising God outright. While they may have received their reward already, our reward is our hope in him. Whatever trials we face, we have confidence knowing that we will never lose Jesus. In him alone we should have satisfaction. †

DAY 144

Mistaken Identity

"In the same way, let your light shine before men, that they may see your good deeds and praise your Father in heaven."

MATTHEW 5:16

You are probably showing enough by now that people around you have begun to feel comfortable asking when you are due, along with other questions about your pregnancy. Some may not approach you yet, apprehensive to ask, not wanting to make a mistake. Six weeks after delivering my twins, my pregnancy pudge had not subsided. While I was pushing my older daughter on a swing, a father smiled and asked me, "So, when are you due?" I smiled, pointed to the stroller holding my "twinfants" and told him, "I'm not. I had twins six weeks ago." Of course, mortified, he stumbled and bumbled, but I assured him it was okay, and I could easily see how the mistake was made.

Christians can also become a case of mistaken identity. When we are ugly, mean, gossiping, and unforgiving, we are hardly the example that Christ calls us to be. Worse yet, if you are identified as a Christian and yet model bad behavior, the case for Christ doesn't seem very appealing. Would someone mistake your identity? †

DAY 145

Brain Waves

"Fix these words of mine in your hearts and minds; tie them as symbols on your hands and bind them on your foreheads. Teach them to your children, talking about them when you sit at home and when you walk along the road, when you lie down and when you get up. Write them on the doorframes of your houses and on your gates. . . ."

DEUTERONOMY 11:18–20

Midway through your pregnancy, your baby has made amazing progress. Brain activity can be measured. Whether you are carrying a boy or a girl, your baby has a mind that is becoming alert, learning, and growing from its environment. For the time being, you can shut out the ugliness of the world. But once your child is born, it is up to you to teach him or her.

Once your baby leaves the protective environment of the womb, what will he or she learn from you? What will you teach your child; what will you impart? You'll teach her by example, but also by what you tell her directly. Will you be ready to teach her everything she needs to know about God? As the Scripture says, "Fix these words of mine in your hearts and minds. . . ." Take some time over the next few weeks to write down some of the beliefs and truths that you most want to fix in her heart and mind. †

DAY 146

A New Look

"You were taught, with regard to your former way of life, to put off your old self, which is being corrupted by its deceitful desires; to be made new in the attitude of your minds. . . ."

EPHESIANS 4:22–23

The big jeans don't fit anymore and the loose, flowing sundress that has doubled as a maternity dress is now too tight. It's time to retire these last holdouts of your former wardrobe. Back pain and pregnancy clumsiness are also probably forcing the high heels to the back of the closet while the tennis shoes and comfy flats find more favor. You are literally putting off the old wardrobe and putting on a new one.

When we become Christians, God asks us to do the same thing. Just as during pregnancy you don't immediately begin to wear maternity clothes but rather add in new items bit by bit, a Christian's walk in sanctification is also ongoing. Under God's direction, you have already put off many of your former ways as you grow in his ways. What is left of your former life? Have you been holding on to a certain area, hoping God doesn't ask you to give it up? Pray for his will to be implemented in every aspect of your life as you walk day by day, growing closer to the person God intends you to be. †

DAY 147

Return to Me

"'Ever since the time of your forefathers you have turned away from my decrees and have not kept them. Return to me, and I will return to you,' says the LORD *Almighty. . . ."*

MALACHI 3:7

Seasons of separateness come for all of us. There are days when it feels like God is really far away. Usually the sense of separation comes because we have created the distance, not him. In the middle of sin, it is hard to go to church, knowing the message might cause conviction. Conviction requires action, a decision either to repent and turn or to continue in sin. Most would rather not approach conviction at all. Church attendance or gathering with fellow Christians becomes sporadic, and people find themselves separated from the fold. Or, when the lines of communication are down, it is difficult to hear what God is trying to say to us. Though the prayers are going up, the conversation is one-way because no time is spent in the Word hearing what God is saying back.

As far as God may feel to you, he hasn't left. Sometimes it just takes us coming back to him to feel his presence. Return to him today. †

Perfect Oneness

"For this reason a man will leave his father and mother and be united to his wife, and they will become one flesh."

GENESIS 2:24

While pregnant with our first child, I worried that making love might somehow be harmful. My husband would try to engage me, yet my mind was so concerned over the welfare of the baby that I wasn't tuned in.

Unless the doctor has specifically instructed you to abstain from intercourse, there is no reason not to enjoy intimacy during this special season. Your baby is nestled in your womb, completely unaware of what is going on and very safely protected. In fact, not only is baby safe, but you may find this a time of increased desire and satisfaction due to the physical changes of pregnancy.

Before the fateful apple tree, intercourse was given to man and woman as a gift that transcends the purpose of reproduction. If you view intercourse as obligatory or somehow sinful or uncomfortable because of your size or worry, release those bondages to God. Focus instead on this wonderful oneness to be shared, the oneness that created your baby and the oneness that is a gift for you and your husband alone. †

DAY 149

Side Sleeping

". . . I ask that we love one another. And this is love: that we walk in obedience to his commands. As you have heard from the beginning, his command is that you walk in love."

2 JOHN 1:5–6

I longed to sleep on my tummy, head flat on the pillow, arms stretched out above me. Besides being impossible once my belly began to bulge, this was a no-no. My second favorite option, flat on my back, was also not advisable. The recommended position on my left side was not how I wanted to sleep. Relief came only with strategically placed pillows and at the point of exhaustion. Though it wasn't my preference, I knew it was best for the baby. For the duration of my pregnancy, it was far better for me to sleep properly, than to sleep comfortably.

Much of our life is spent the same way; we do things the right way even though we may not feel like it, knowing it is for our own benefit. God's instructions and commands are not meant to hinder or control us. Rather, they are intended to bless us, ensuring we live a life that will yield blessing and satisfaction rather than the hurt and pain that are consequences of sin. †

DAY 150

Stalled

"A patient man has great understanding, but a quick-tempered man displays folly."

PROVERBS 14:29

Like a car stuck smack in the middle of a long line of traffic, you might feel stalled right now. You've come a long way since your pregnancy started, but the end isn't in sight. You feel like nothing is moving, even in the restroom, where constipation is one of the plagues of pregnancy.

While high-fiber foods or supplements can jump-start a stalled digestive system, what do you do when you feel like you are spiritually stalled in a pregnancy traffic jam? As on the road, you can get impatient and annoyed, which only enhances your frustration. Or, you can choose to enjoy the moment, regardless of the circumstances. Listen to the music of your life; enjoy the little blessings that are all around you. Take your eyes off of the long wait and enjoy your surroundings. What if you weren't waiting right now? You might be rushing to the hospital for preterm labor. Patience now means you have more time to bond, to plan, to prepare your heart and home for Baby's arrival. †

DAY 151

A Lost Child

"And if he finds it, I tell you the truth, he is happier about that one sheep than about the ninety-nine that did not wander off."
MATTHEW 18:13

Over the last few months, you've formed a bond of love with your child. Already you can't imagine life without him and will do anything to preserve his life and keep him close to you.

Nothing instills more panic in a mother than the thought of a lost child. Once, on the way to school, one of my toddler twins became separated from me. One moment he was safely holding my hand; the next, he had completely vanished. The panic intensified with every passing moment. Suddenly every person, and each car in the car pool, was potentially carrying my baby away from me. When he was found, sheer relief and joy consumed me. He was lost and had come back again. My arms never wanted to let him go.

That is the way Christ feels about us. We were lost, a sheep separated from the fold. He loves us so much that he died in order to bring us back, to restore us. He loved you so much that he would rather die than face eternal separation from you. Because of him, we are no longer lost. †

DAY 152

My Shepherd

"The Lord *is my shepherd, I shall not be in want."*

Psalm 23:1

As one who was like a sheep and rescued, you now have a Shepherd. You do not go through life alone, isolated, unprotected, and unguarded from the dangers around you. You are part of God's fold and have the Almighty as your Shepherd. Psalm 23 is a beautiful reminder of what our life can look like when God is our Shepherd. In him we have rest, we have peace, and we have restoration. Though we face trials and even death, we do not have to have fear, because we have him who comforts us.

We can utterly and completely rely on him, depending on him every day of our life. He goes before us in every interaction, even with our enemies, and he gives us favor. Because of him, we can say with confidence just as the psalmist David said, "Surely goodness and love will follow me all the days of my life, and I will dwell in the house of the Lord forever" (Psalm 23:6). He is your Father. He is your Shepherd. He is your God. †

DAY 153

Unspoken Words

". . . Paul sent for the disciples and, after encouraging them, said good-by and set out for Macedonia. He traveled through that area, speaking many words of encouragement to the people. . . ."

ACTS 20:1–2

Within every relationship, there is a finite window of opportunity. When the window is open, we have an opportunity to tell that person how we feel, expressing how much we love them and what they have meant to us. At some point the window will close. Whether through death, divorce, or distance, eventually there will come a time when the window closes, shutting off the opportunity to speak those important words.

Every day God puts people into your life that you value, whether precious friends or family members. Who are those special people in your life right now, the ones sharing this special season of pregnancy? Who are the people who will play an important role in the life of this child? Have you told them lately what they mean to you, what a blessing they have been to you? At some point, the window of opportunity will close and you will be unable to share with them. Today, while your windows are open, tell the ones in your life what they mean to you, how thankful you are for them, and how much you love them. Don't live a life of unspoken words. †

DAY 154

An Authentic Life

"Rather, as servants of God we commend ourselves in every way: in great endurance; in troubles, hardships and distresses; in beatings, imprisonments and riots; in hard work, sleepless nights and hunger; in purity, understanding, patience and kindness; in the Holy Spirit and in sincere love; in truthful speech and in the power of God; with weapons of righteousness in the right hand and in the left; through glory and dishonor, bad report and good report; genuine, yet regarded as impostors. . . ."

2 CORINTHIANS 6:4–8

Now that you're enrobed in maternity clothes and your expanded belly is evident to all, you might feel authentically pregnant. While you've felt pregnant all along, these emerging signs give a sense of credibility, like you can now call yourself a full-fledged member of the "I'm expecting" club.

Spiritually, authenticity is just as important. God desires us to not just call ourselves Christians, but to really experience Christ in the seasons of drought and in plenty. Having an authentic walk means that God truly does hold the number one, authoritative position in your life. As a result, everything in your life has been transformed in realignment with him. Having an authentic life translates into believing that each and every day, your life is lived on the premise of his promises. You are genuinely his; is your life lived genuinely for him? †

DAY 155

Just Like Him

"'I will be a Father to you, and you will be my sons and daughters,' says the LORD *Almighty."*

2 CORINTHIANS 6:18

I have the privilege of holding the most important title of my life: mom. I will always be my children's mother from the day I became pregnant until the day my children pass. I am painfully aware that every time I sin, every time I say or do something, I am modeling behavior that my children may one day emulate. Of all the things I will always be to them, the one thing I will never be is their father.

Every day I watch my children seek their father's approval. They want to be just like him. He is their earthly representation of who God is. They strive to receive his praise, his validation, his approval. Because they want to be just like Dad, I pray that he is ever growing closer to the image of his Father.

For your child, your husband will hold that same importance. As your baby is growing, pray for the father, that each day he would grow closer to God, giving those innocent eyes a living example of their heavenly Father above. †

Practice

". . . 'Now the dwelling of God is with men, and he will live with them. They will be his people, and God himself will be with them and be their God. He will wipe every tear from their eyes. There will be no more death or mourning or crying or pain, for the old order of things has passed away.'"

REVELATION 21:3–4

Every so often you probably feel a tightening across your lower abdomen. It tightens, becomes rock hard, and then relaxes again. Braxton Hicks contractions are a normal, healthy way that your body prepares for delivery. Practicing for the big event is smart. In the weeks ahead you'll practice breathing, perhaps practice changing diapers, or other baby-care techniques.

Spiritually we practice, too. How we glorify God in our life here on Earth is practice for the main event of our hope everlasting. Just as we can't comprehend the joy of holding the baby until she arrives, we can't begin to understand what glory awaits us in the kingdom to come. Until then, we have opportunities to experience the everlasting. We have hope through the Holy Spirit, we get to join with the angels in praising through song and words, and we get to talk through our prayer life. Thank you, God, that we can practice now for eternity with you. †

DAY 157

Fanning the Flame

"For this reason I remind you to fan into flame the gift of God, which is in you through the laying on of my hands. For God did not give us a spirit of timidity, but a spirit of power, of love and of self-discipline."

2 TIMOTHY 1:6–7

Leg cramps are common in pregnancy. For me, it would feel like a knife stabbing my calves. I'd be blissfully sleeping when my muscles would tighten and contract, sending shooting pain through my legs. Your body nourishes the baby first, depleting its own supply of minerals. The resulting deficit causes the leg cramps. My husband would fetch a banana for me in the night, hoping that the potassium in the banana would replenish my supply and ease my pain.

Throughout my pregnancy, my husband was always willing to bring me bananas or a glass of water. Afterward, when I was exhausted from nursing, he would gently change the baby's diaper and carry our little bundle to me so I could get a few minutes of sleep.

So often it is the little gestures of kindness that fan the flames of the relationship during the mundane moments of life. Your husband has probably been doing more little things for you lately, a demonstration of his love for you. How about him? Are you fanning the flame as well, showing your love for him in little ways? †

Feeling Moody

"Rejoice in the Lord *always. I will say it again: Rejoice! Let your gentleness be evident to all. The* Lord *is near."*

Philippians 4:4–5

Just when you thought you'd returned to normal, something sparked your anger. Maybe you asked your husband to go to a doctor's appointment with you, but he was unable to attend due to work. Or maybe it was something really minor like the way he gave his attention to the television rather than you. Usually, the grumpiness is over nothing—insignificant little events that otherwise would be no big deal—but when your body is awash in pregnancy hormones, everything takes on new significance. It's all part of the process of your body preparing to give birth. So when you start to feel upset and can't understand it, focus instead on the preparation for the upcoming birth.

It's good preparation for the months ahead when other things will make you grumpy, like lack of sleep and unending laundry. Practice focusing on what is good. Look to the Lord, not just as the provider of your physical needs, but also as the provider of your spiritual and emotional needs. He is able to give you peace. Cast your eyes on him, not on the details derailing your focus. †

DAY 159

In the Context of Christ

"But even if you should suffer for what is right, you are blessed. 'Do not fear what they fear; do not be frightened.' But in your hearts set apart Christ as LORD. *Always be prepared to give an answer to everyone who asks you to give the reason for the hope that you have. But do this with gentleness and respect, keeping a clear conscience, so that those who speak maliciously against your good behavior in Christ may be ashamed of their slander."*

1 PETER 3:14–16

Context makes all the difference. If you wear shorts and a T-shirt on a sunny, hot day, it's no big deal right? But it could cause an uproar if you wore that outfit to a formal summertime wedding. Clothes should fit not only the weather, but the occasion. Right now you are living in the context of pregnancy; your condition determines the type of clothes you wear, what food you eat, how strenuously you exercise, and more.

As a Christian, you are called to live a life in the context of Christ, rather than the context of the world. It's a life set apart, one that does not look like everyone else's, but is lived according to God's words and purpose. In the context of Christ, Christians stand strong in adversity, trials, upsets, and defeats, knowing that their hope is not on what today brings, but is the eternal hope of tomorrow. Are you living your life in the context of Christ? Return to living in his context, in his grace, in his love, and in his purpose. †

DAY 160

Bank of Christ

"For it is by grace you have been saved, through faith—and this not from yourselves, it is the gift of God—not by works, so that no one can boast."

EPHESIANS 2:8–9

Many people operate with a sense that admission to heaven works like a bank, believing that their abundant deposits of good deeds, well wishes, and virtuous living will cover their withdrawals when they sin. If they make enough deposits by going to church, volunteering, being good, or not breaking the law, the merits of their actions will wipe away their sin; surely they are good enough to go to heaven.

Virtue, good deeds, and an honorable character are wonderful attributes, but when it comes to heaven, they don't count. Those deposits in the bank account of your life should be more like earned interest that naturally accrues because the perfect deposit of Christ resides in your heart. Just one sin causes spiritual bankruptcy. Just one sin separates us from God. No matter how many "good" deposits there are, even one "bad" withdrawal creates eternal separation from God, and Christ is the only redemption. Do you have the perfect deposit of Christ in your life? †

Costly Grace

"In him we have redemption through his blood, the forgiveness of sins, in accordance with the riches of God's grace that he lavished on us with all wisdom and understanding."

EPHESIANS 1:7–8

The costs add up: doctor or midwife fees, maternity clothes, hospital bills, items for the nursery, baby supplies. Though creating this life may not have cost you anything, ensuring it is brought into the world is expensive! Grace is much the same way. Though God's grace is free for the asking, available to all, the price wasn't cheap.

For us to be called sons of God, to be able to share eternity in heaven with the Most High, required a costly redemption from our sins. We have no way to pay the debt. Yet, it is available as a free gift. It can't be earned by making donations or sacrificing personal possessions. It doesn't even cost us jail time or community service hours. Redemption, the ability to have His grace extended to us, was paid by no less than the blood of Jesus. In him, we can find forgiveness. †

DAY 162

Made Alive

"As for you, you were dead in your transgressions and sins, in which you used to live when you followed the ways of this world and of the ruler of the kingdom of the air, the spirit who is now at work in those who are disobedient. All of us also lived among them at one time, gratifying the cravings of our sinful nature and following its desires and thoughts. Like the rest, we were by nature objects of wrath."

EPHESIANS 2:1–3

From the moment of conception, your body has been working hard in the miraculous process of making a baby. Moment by moment, your baby is being formed, growing, and developing, so that at the point of delivery, she will be able to take her first breaths and survive outside the nourishment of your womb.

Once you made the decision to follow Christ, though physically alive, you passed from a spiritual death to a new life in him. By placing your trust and faith in him, you received the free gift of salvation. Because of his great love, you have been snatched from the grip of the evil one and given life everlasting. Despite this transformation, there are still some days when you feel like you need the rejuvenation of Christ. Like a glass that has been dropped, shattered into a thousand pieces, you need his love to make you whole. He is the only one who is able to take our broken hearts and our weary souls and breathe new life into them. Take a breath of Jesus today, allowing him to restore your soul. †

DAY 163

Too Big or Too Small?

"I pray that out of his glorious riches he may strengthen you with power through his Spirit in your inner being, so that Christ may dwell in your hearts through faith. . . ."

EPHESIANS 3:16–17

A lot of belly analysis is probably occurring right now. Some days you think your tummy looks too small, causing worry or concern. Other times you wonder, "How can I possibly have sixteen weeks to go?" Almost every woman has these thoughts during pregnancy. Belly shapes and sizes are as varied among women as hairstyle, height, and bone structure. What is normal for one woman isn't necessarily normal for you.

Sometimes it's easy to feel like your faith is too small. As much as you want to believe God's promises, your eyes see the reality around you and overwhelming hopelessness instead. On days when you really see God moving, it is easier to have huge faith, faith that is punctuated by the presence of his promises. Yet, faith shouldn't be contingent on circumstances, but consistent in seasons of drought and plenty. Do you feel like you are lacking in faith? Ask for it. Don't be embarrassed or ashamed, but instead ask that your faith will grow, each day more than the last and tomorrow's greater than today. †

Eyes That See and Ears That Hear

"For this people's heart has become calloused; they hardly hear with their ears, and they have closed their eyes. Otherwise they might see with their eyes, hear with their ears, understand with their hearts and turn, and I would heal them. But blessed are your eyes because they see, and your ears because they hear."

MATTHEW 13:15–16

When asked if they want a boy or a girl, most women respond with only one hope, a healthy baby. As soon as the baby is born, moms instinctively inspect their child, counting toes, kissing fingers, talking to the little open ears.

Most babies enter into this world in perfect physical condition. When there are special needs such as Down syndrome, hearing impairment, or blindness, God still gives us everything we need. He asks that we have eyes that would see. To be able to "see" doesn't necessarily mean having eyes that physically see, but having a spirit that is receptive to seeing what God would have us live and do.

God also asks that we have ears that hear. As a child of two completely hearing-impaired parents, I am acutely aware of how much the deaf "hear," though audible sounds may escape them. When you choose to go through life seeing and hearing regardless of the physical equipment you may have, you will have a life of blessing. Have eyes that see and ears that hear. †

DAY 165

Warning Signs

"To whom can I speak and give warning? Who will listen to me? Their ears are closed so they cannot hear. The word of the LORD *is offensive to them; they find no pleasure in it."*

JEREMIAH 6:10

I'd already been hospitalized for a week and was safely at home on full bed rest. Beside my bed was a contraction monitor that would send a report to a nurse every few hours. Based upon the reading each day, she'd determine whether I could remain home or return to the hospital. One day the report indicated that the situation was worsening. I was sent back to the hospital, where I remained until the birth of my twins.

In pregnancy there are warning signs when the body is no longer cooperating with the pregnancy—contractions or pressure signaling the onset of preterm labor, or swelling that could indicate pre-eclampsia. In your spiritual walk there are also warning signs that you are becoming distant from God. They take the form of little sins like gossiping or telling a little white lie. Or there could be bigger signs. Are you unable to remember the last time you picked up the Bible? Just as carefully as you monitor warning signs in pregnancy, monitor the warning signs of your spiritual life, too. †

DAY 166

Standing in Awe

"Therefore, since we are receiving a kingdom that cannot be shaken, let us be thankful, and so worship God acceptably with reverence and awe. . . ."

HEBREWS 12:28

Remember the awe and wonder of the first week of pregnancy, of the miracle that was growing inside of you? Now that you are safely in the middle of the second trimester, has the awe of the pregnancy worn off a bit? It's no longer new. It may feel a little commonplace, as though you've been pregnant your whole life and you're not sure how or when you could ever feel not pregnant again.

Complacency can be a danger of living a blessed life. When you first moved into your home, it may have felt like a castle, but now it is routine, maybe even cramped, and you may feel a twinge of desire for something new. Salvation is much the same way. In the beginning, the realization of salvation inspires a desire to share the greatness of God with the whole world. But after a few years, the fire may have died down. Rekindle the embers of your awe and gratitude. Restore the fire of thankfulness in your heart. Stand in awe of God. †

DAY 167

Too Little or Too Much?

"At the present time your plenty will supply what they need, so that in turn their plenty will supply what you need. Then there will be equality, as it is written: 'He who gathered much did not have too much, and he who gathered little did not have too little.'"

2 CORINTHIANS 8:14–15

Have you figured out the magic formula of just how many receiving blankets, onesies, and newborn-sized outfits you will need for this baby? Does your child need two hooded towels or twelve? Certainly, you want a supply ample enough to ensure that you aren't running a load of laundry after every diaper change. But, at the same time you don't want more than you can possibly use or even store. With the birth of our daughter, the urge to buy cute baby girl clothes was irresistable. We could have outfitted her in a new dress every day of her life and not depleted her supply. Yet, when it came to the bigger sizes we found ourselves hitting the store aisles again.

Isn't it nice that in Christ we don't have to worry about how much or how little he loves us? His love is complete, demonstrated by his death on the cross. Though each of us falls short of his perfect standard, once "in Him," we receive the full provision of his love and grace. Because of Christ we each have perfect Providence. †

DAY 168

Prayerful Preparation

"Yet give attention to your servant's prayer and his plea for mercy, O LORD my God. Hear the cry and the prayer that your servant is praying in your presence."

2 CHRONICLES 6:19

This time of pregnancy is a perfect time to slowly but surely make progress on your nursery. Though painting is off-limits for mom, there isn't any reason why you can't help fix up the nursery in other ways. Before my first baby was born, I would go into the room we'd prepared for him; sit on the rocking chair with my hands on my belly; and pray for him, for the delivery, for his life, who he was going to become, and for us as parents. I loved sitting in the rocker, imagining the months ahead when I would not be holding my belly, but my precious, beautiful baby boy.

I haven't stopped praying for him, even though he is no longer a tiny infant, but a big eleven-year-old boy. Though I can't hold him in my arms, I still pray for him constantly, knowing God is preparing him for the day at hand and the days to come. †

DAY 169

Viability

". . . your eyes saw my unformed body. All the days ordained for me were written in your book before one of them came to be."

Psalm 139:16

Your baby has reached an important milestone; he is considered legally and medically viable. Simply stated, if your baby were born today, your child could survive outside the womb, though serious medical intervention would be required. Of course, as a mother, you are anxious to see your child, but you want to wait as long as possible, until the baby is full term, before it is delivered. Each day the baby spends in the womb gives her strength, protection, and time to grow.

To you, this baby was fully alive from the moment you discovered you were pregnant. To God, this child was known before he was even created in your womb. Before this child was even formed, God knew the number of hairs he would have, the number of days he would spend in your womb, and every thought that would cross his mind. As you pray, watching the clock and calendar for the arrival of this precious life, know that God also knows your child's birthday, the exact moment he will make his entry. God's knowledge is complete, lacking nothing. †

Feed My Sheep

". . . Peter was hurt because Jesus asked him the third time, 'Do you love me?' He said, 'LORD, you know all things; you know that I love you.' Jesus said, 'Feed my sheep.'"

JOHN 21:17–18

Between you and Baby, there's a lot of feeding going on. You're taking in extra calories in order to supply the nutritional needs of your baby and yourself. You've also spent time spiritually feeding your body by spending time in the Word, praying, and reading this devotional. What else could you feed right now? Others.

In the book of John, God's Word is clear: if we love Christ, we are to feed his sheep. That may mean literally inviting those people to dinner, to share a meal in your home for a time of fellowship. It also means feeding them with love, being a palpable representation of Christ. When we extend Christ's love to others, we have the privilege of being utilized for his glory, taking part in an eternal miracle. Just as he rescued you from the fold, bringing you safely back to him, he desires that every lost person would also return to safety. Have you been feeding his sheep? †

DAY 171

The Power of Two

". . . Then Jesus went around teaching from village to village. Calling the Twelve to him, he sent them out two by two and gave them authority over evil spirits."

MARK 6:6–7

God did not make a mistake in giving a baby both a mother and a father. Having two parents to shape and care for a child provides a unique and far-reaching love. The power of two in all things is immense. In the Creation, God made both man and woman so man would not be alone but would have a companion. When two or more are gathered, there is power in their prayer—Matthew 18:20 says, "For where two or three come together in my name, there am I with them." When Jesus sent out the twelve disciples, he sent them in groups of two.

Why two? Because when one is alone, there is inherent danger: that person stands alone, isolated, removed from the safety of others. When one stands alone, there is no one to help her when she falls. In two there is strength. In the days ahead your helper, your husband will help strengthen, encourage, and assist you. Even if you face motherhood without a partner, God will put people in your life so that you do not stand alone, whether trusted friend, family member, or sister. Thankfully, in parenthood, you do not face the road alone. †

DAY 172

Known by Actions

"At Caesarea there was a man named Cornelius, a centurion in what was known as the Italian Regiment. He and all his family were devout and God-fearing; he gave generously to those in need and prayed to God regularly."

ACTS 10:1–2

We are all aware that we are not alone in this world, that each of our actions affects others. Every time you attend a medical examination, you are known by your doctor for your persistence in questions, your gentleness in spirit, or your impatience for Baby to arrive. Our reputations are built on our actions, whether we are successful, reliable, scatter-brained, or careless. How you do something defines you as much as what you do.

Cornelius was known as God-fearing, someone who gave to those in need and prayed to God regularly. How are you known? Is it how you want to be known? Have a vision of the person you want to be and begin to take steps toward becoming that person. Whether you realize it or not, you are already known by your actions. †

DAY 173

In You

"Be my rock of refuge, to which I can always go; give the command to save me, for you are my rock and my fortress."

PSALM 71:3

Pregnancy books were one of my favorite resources during pregnancy. I would feel a pang and immediately turn through the pages to discern what I was feeling. Before long, I knew instinctively where to flip in the book, knowing its words cover to cover. Often, before I sought God, I sought those pages. Then I realized that I was putting more trust in those words than in God's Word. Though I needed medical advice, I also needed God's peace and wisdom. Though I needed to reassure myself that I was normal, I also needed to know what he was saying to me in those circumstances.

Do you find yourself in the same situation? God is our rock, our refuge that is eternal, always present, and immediately accessible. Whether we are driving in the car, removed from the resources of the Internet and books, or in the middle of a doctor's office when a flag indicates something might be wrong, he is there. Let him be your rock today. Put your trust in him. †

DAY 174

What You Can

"'How many loaves do you have?' he asked. 'Go and see.' When they found out, they said, 'Five—and two fish.'"

MARK 6:38

Pregnancy is a time of introspection and thought, preparing your heart and body for parenting. During pregnancy, you may not exactly feel like you can do a whole lot for God, but in every season of our life, God just asks that we be willing to share what we have.

When Jesus fed the 5,000, he didn't simply create the food out of thin air, but allowed the people to be involved in the miracle. Though they only had five loaves of bread and two fish to offer a crowd of 5,000, God used what they had and performed a miracle. He does the same with you. Whatever it is, God asks that you be ready to use what you have. Don't focus on the equipment you don't have, feeling paralyzed by your shortcomings. Instead, look at the talents, skills, knowledge, and abilities you do have. He won't ask you to do something you have not been equipped to do. Only one thing is required: a willing and receptive heart. †

DAY 175

A Gentle Spirit

"Let your gentleness be evident to all. The LORD *is near."*

PHILIPPIANS 4:5

Going to the grocery store while pregnant with twins was not exactly something I enjoyed. Within my family, I am notorious for having a knack for always choosing the slowest checkout line and never finding a close parking space. My older two kids would be restless to leave, wanting to purchase everything in sight, while we'd be stuck in line as prices were checked, coupons shuffled, and cash-register tape replaced. When I was asked for the twelfth time if they could "pleeeease" get a candy bar, my response was not exactly gentle.

Grumpiness rather than gentleness is a natural reaction in pregnancy when you feel big, clumsy, tired, and drained. All it takes is someone's careless comment or a child's whining to set it off. Yet, God calls us to be gentle to all, not just when you are in a good mood and just to those people whom you like. *All* means *everyone,* even unlikable people in unpleasant situations. †

DAY 176

Don't Give Up

"Devote yourselves to prayer, being watchful and thankful."

COLOSSIANS 4:2

When there is danger or turbulence in our lives, our fear prompts us to seek out God and pray. But when everything is going great, the requests don't come to our hearts and minds as quickly. When pregnancy is smooth sailing, it is easy to forget to pray. The baby is moving regularly, doctor visits are routine, and no warning signs have surfaced. Perhaps in your marriage, things are smooth too; your career is advancing, your relationships with your family and friends are solid, and life is good. It is easy to become complacent in prayer when you don't have a pressing need.

When life is in a season of ease, focus your prayers on offering thanksgiving for what you have. Infuse your prayers with praise and requests for protection, continued health, and continued blessing. Don't allow the ease of today to hinder your prayer life. †

DAY 177

Certainty of Christ

"But the fruit of the Spirit is love, joy, peace, patience, kindness, goodness, faithfulness, gentleness and self-control. Against such things there is no law."

Galations 5:22–23

"When are you due?" "What are you having?" "Are you having a C-section?" "Will you breast-feed?" You are probably getting a little tired of perfect strangers inquiring about the most intimate details of your life. Because you have this protruding belly, a sure sign of the pregnancy within, people are drawn to you and feel at ease—even placing their hands on your tummy to feel the baby.

Christians also tend to play a similar role in the community. Because of how you have shown love or helped in a community, you may be the first one they seek for help in times of turmoil. Though the signs you display are not as obvious as your belly, you have other fruits confirming your faith. You have the fruits of the spirit: patience, kindness, gentleness, being slow to anger and abundant with love. The fruits of our lives bear witness to who we are, giving clear and evident reminders to all about whom we love and what we believe. Are you bearing fruit? †

DAY 178

Important Ingredients

"As you do not know the path of the wind, or how the body is formed in a mother's womb, so you cannot understand the work of God, the Maker of all things."

Ecclesiastes 11:5

This week a very important job is underway in the baby's lungs. Surfactant is being produced and lining the lungs. It's an important substance, allowing the lungs to fill with air, rather than being stuck together inside. God provides the baby with everything it needs to thrive—the amniotic sac, the umbilical cord, the placenta. He produces all the important ingredients for life, ensuring that the smallest details are attended to, giving us everything we need to live.

He is concerned with not only the big life-support system of creation, but the intricate details as well. Each person is crafted with unique talents and abilities as different and varied as any two lives are. Though all four of my children are born of the same parents, and two of them are identical twins with matching DNA, all four are uniquely talented. Though they may overlap in interests, each excels independently and uniquely. As God uniquely crafts your child, pray to have eyes open to the gifts he gives them, and a heart that helps develop the children in the way God intended. †

DAY 179

The Perfect One

"But my dove, my perfect one, is unique, the only daughter of her mother, the favorite of the one who bore her. The maidens saw her and called her blessed; the queens and concubines praised her."

SONG OF SONGS 6:9

He or she may be growing in utero right now, soon to be conceived, or have been alive for a while. Somewhere out there exists the person your child will eventually come to love and to marry. In Song of Songs, the beloved describes his bride as his perfect one. He does not call her perfect, but perfect for him. You are partnered to the perfect one for you; your husband is not a perfect person, just as he is partnered to you despite your imperfections.

Pray now that your child will have the discernment to end relationships that are unhealthy, that he would have a heart that leads him to the one God has purposed for him, and that he would not take a detour and settle for less on the road to companionship. Pray for his future spouse, that she, too, would wait for the one God has created for her, that her heart would be molded to Christ, and that she would be protected and guarded throughout her childhood. †

Who Was, Who Is, and Who Is to Come

"'I am the Alpha and the Omega,' says the LORD *God, 'who is, and who was, and who is to come, the Almighty.'"*

REVELATION 1:8

Everything we do is measured in increments of time. How many days until your baby is born . . . how many minutes until dinnertime . . . how many years you'll spend on this earth . . . Our society operates on the fundamental basis of time, running by clocks and calendars. To grasp eternity—the concept of "always was and always will be"—is beyond our scope of imagination.

Time never passes with ease, usually passing too slowly when we are in pain and too quickly when we are rejoicing. As you long to hold your baby, anticipating her delivery day, you may feel time has never passed so slowly. Yet, by this time next year, you will wonder where the last twelve months have gone! Because the speed of the clock always surprises us, time alone suggests that we were not created for this temporal existence, but for God's eternal presence. God is timeless. God always was. He is now. And he is the One to come. He is Alpha, the beginning, and he is Omega, the end. All things in heaven and Earth begin and end with him. One day we will be reunited with our Father, the one who was, who is, and who is to come. †

DAY 181

Hurting Hearts

"The poor and needy search for water, but there is none; their tongues are parched with thirst. But I the Lord *will answer them; I, the God of Israel, will not forsake them."*

Isaiah 41:17

I was gripped with fear. My knuckles grasped the rails of my hospital bed as IV lines dripped terbutaline into my veins. The words "We only have a fifty percent chance of stopping your labor" ran through my head over and over again. My babies, my precious babies, were in grave danger, and I was utterly powerless to help them. "Oh, Jesus," was all I could manage; I was so wracked with worry that the little lives might face hospitalization, impairment, or even death if born too early.

Sometimes we are so gripped with fear or need that we are like the poor and needy, so thirsty and parched our lips can't verbalize the requests of our spirit. In those moments, God doesn't pause, waiting to intercede until we specify our request with the right words. He knows what you need, when you need it. Even when you are too paralyzed to ask, he hears you. He is your Father who loves you in the moment you are in.

My labor miraculously stopped. God had heard my heart. †

DAY 182

To See the Light

"When he looks at me, he sees the one who sent me. I have come into the world as a light, so that no one who believes in me should stay in darkness."

JOHN 12:45–46

Your baby is already receptive to light. If you were to shine a light on your belly, baby might respond, perhaps turning away from the light to shield its eyes, or turning toward the light in curiosity. Even now, within your womb, baby is learning to differentiate between light and darkness, before he has even seen the light of the world.

As a believer in Christ, you have experienced the light of the world. You know what it is to stand in lightness and not to live in darkness any longer. You have experienced the joy of walking in forgiveness, the gift of grace and a second birth. Your heart is full of thanksgiving for the light that was given to us through Jesus's death and resurrection. You no longer have to feel ashamed, condemned, or unworthy, because he has called you his own and you stand blameless before him. Though you will share physical light and darkness, morning and night, with your child, you will also share the eternal light. †

The Touch of His Robe

"He said to her, 'Daughter, your faith has healed you. Go in peace and be freed from your suffering.'"

MARK 5:34

She had been sick for twelve years. Though she had sought remedies, her bleeding body received no relief. One day she heard about Jesus coming through her town and went to find him. Knowing how busy he was, she did not seek to take his time or to keep him from his work. She just wanted his touch, believing it could heal her.

As the crowd approached, she boldly reached out and touched his garment. Though he was constantly handled by the crowds, he discerned her touch as different. He asked, "Who touched me?" (Mark 5:31). Because of his healing power, the woman suffered no more. Coupled with her faith, the touch of his cloak was enough to bring healing.

You have this Jesus too, interceding on your behalf with the Father. If this pregnancy has brought medical complications for you or your child, you may be wondering if and when God will bring healing. We don't know why sometimes God heals on earth or chooses to give a heavenly healing, but we do know his will is perfect. Just as his touch was perfect for her restoration, it is also perfect for yours. Receive his healing touch today. †

DAY 184

House of God

"So I rebuked the officials and asked them, 'Why is the house of God neglected?' Then I called them together and stationed them at their posts."

NEHEMIAH 13:11

As the day of your baby's arrival comes closer, your body, spirit, and home are growing more ready. You're probably readying your house so that no detail is overlooked or neglected when your baby comes into your home.

God also desires that we do not neglect his house. Just as your house requires everyone to help out with maintenance and cleaning, the house of God requires that all pitch in too. Do you have a church family? As a believer, you belong in a church body where you can be fed spiritually and you can help feed others as well. Have you been contributing to the house of God with your attendance, tithing, and support?

Members of the body of Christ should make it a priority to participate in a church family as directed by God. After your baby is born, it will be much more difficult to begin to do these things if you aren't already in the practice of doing so. Ensure both the home where you reside and your house of God are not in neglect. †

DAY 185

Loving Hands

"For the LORD *is the great God, the great King above all gods. In his hand are the depths of the earth, and the mountain peaks belong to him."*

PSALM 95:3–4

In a few weeks, my brother-in-law will become a father for the first time. As the months have passed, we've watched him engage in the pregnancy, accompanying his wife to doctor visits or feeling Baby's kicks through his wife's belly. I'm not even sure he notices it, how often he gently places his hand there, a connection to the daughter he has not yet held. As his hand rests there, hoping to feel movement, a slight smile graces his face though he is fully engaged in conversation. The connection and love between father and daughter is being created before she has even left the womb.

We know our heavenly Father, too, by the evidence of him all around us. We see his glory in his creations. We see the depth of his love in the blood of Jesus. We see his provision in our blessings. God's evidence of his love is abundant. Look at your life today and see how he has been placing his loving hands on your life. †

DAY 186

My Daily Bread

"He humbled you, causing you to hunger and then feeding you with manna, which neither you nor your fathers had known, to teach you that man does not live on bread alone but on every word that comes from the mouth of the LORD."

DEUTERONOMY 8:3

The children of Israel left the abundance of Egypt for a life where they were completely dependent on God. They had been rescued from the grip of slavery but found that they were nomads in the desert, relying moment by moment on God's provision of food and safety. They grumbled against Moses and God, complaining even to the point of saying they were better off as slaves in Egypt. But God did not deliver them to the desert to leave them to die.

The Israelites expected an immediate reprieve, a land of blessing. Instead they had to go through a period of trial to learn faith and test their hearts. In the desert, God provided them daily bread from heaven, manna.

Right now, the demands of impending parenthood and increased responsibilities might begin to overwhelm you. You may have thought that by this time in your life, you would have more savings, a bigger home, or a larger salary. Just as God provided for the Israelites, he will provide for you. Allow him to be your daily bread. †

DAY 187

Feeling Ugly

"Your beauty should not come from outward adornment, such as braided hair and the wearing of gold jewelry and fine clothes. Instead, it should be that of your inner self, the unfading beauty of a gentle and quiet spirit, which is of great worth in God's sight."

1 PETER 3:3–4

With each passing week I felt like my ugly factor was increasing. I would see less of the person I used to look like and look more like a balloon ready to pop. I would try to fix my hair or wear flattering clothes. The only perk of having such a big belly was that my thighs looked small in contrast. I certainly did not feel attractive or pretty.

However, my husband seemed oblivious to my puffy face and legs and bloated belly. He continued to remark that he thought I looked nice and would pay me compliments like I was the prettiest pregnant person he had ever seen.

Women are beautiful regardless of age, body shape, or uterus size. We can have a beautiful spirit that infuses everything we say and do. A woman with a gentle spirit is much more attractive than a woman who has outer beauty but attacks with words and attitude. Even as you feel ugly, you can be the most beautiful woman in the world. †

DAY 188

Support Systems

"Joanna the wife of Cuza, the manager of Herod's household; Susanna; and many others. These women were helping to support them out of their own means."

LUKE 8:3

When my oldest son was born, we were covered with backup support. Not only was my husband off from work, but I also had my parents and in-laws at my immediate disposal. It was wonderful to have help with meals and cleaning up, and, of course, there was never a shortage of helping hands to hold our precious little one. The only drawback to so many offers of help was sharing him with other arms.

Have you begun to line up help? Deciding ahead of time how you want help will ensure that you obtain effective helpers. Will you need assistance with other children, or will you need help with household duties or meals so that you can focus your efforts on caring for the baby?

God's given you friends and family for support. Don't deprive yourself of this blessing by refusing their help at this time. A rested mother and an organized home make for a happier family. Don't be afraid to ask for help, and don't be ashamed to receive it. Allow others to share in this special time in your life. †

DAY 189

A Heavy Burden

"Take my yoke upon you and learn from me, for I am gentle and humble in heart, and you will find rest for your souls. For my yoke is easy and my burden is light."

MATTHEW 11:29–30

During the last month of my twin pregnancy, I became exponentially bigger each day. When their birth day arrived, I delivered Jon first as the other doctors held James firmly in place to keep him from turning. The relief as the weight of their bodies was lifted from my body was incredible.

I was struck by the physical weight of those two boys, and how loaded down I felt during those last days. How must Jesus have felt carrying the burden of mankind's sin on his shoulders? How heavy was the weight of sin, pressing him down, attempting to defeat him at every turn? The only way to combat this literal weight of the world was through prayer, talking to his father, seeking his will. In these last days of pregnancy, you, too, can find a reprieve from the weight you are carrying. In him, find rest for your soul. †

THIRD TRIMESTER

Finishing Touches

Introduction to the Third Trimester

The third trimester, the final stretch leading up to the grand finale of pregnancy, is a time of mixed feelings. Physically, you may feel fatigued, engorged, cumbersome, and uncomfortable. As your baby grows larger within your womb, he or she puts strain on your innards, kicking your bladder, poking your ribs, and constricting your lungs. Baby may get more rambunctious in the beginning of the third trimester—the internal gymnastics can be quite comical—but will probably settle down as the weeks pass and the space in the womb becomes more cramped. Emotionally, you're full of joyous anticipation, knowing that your baby will arrive soon, but the feeling may also be a bit bittersweet because your pregnancy experience will come to a conclusion soon.

Where the second trimester is all about baby practicing for life outside the womb, the third trimester is a time for mom's body to practice for bringing baby into the world. Practice contractions, called Braxton Hicks, are an inconsistent, painless tightening of the uterine muscles, sort of a warm-up for labor. Meanwhile, your hormones prompt your ligaments and joints to soften and relax. While this will make it easier for your baby to pass through your pelvis at delivery, it can cause backaches and hip pain. Your breasts are getting ready too, producing colostrum, a precursor to the breast milk that provides nourishment and immunity to your baby after birth. The placenta begins to produce and pass along antibodies that will offer protection and immunity to your baby against the dangers of the outside world.

So what's Baby up to during the last trimester? He opens his eyes, which have been fused shut, and is sensitive to his environment, both inside and outside the womb. His organs continue to mature and develop, getting ready to function after birth. Most importantly, he devotes his energy to growing and gaining weight.

When the time comes, contractions will thin and dilate the cervix, opening up the passageway for baby to transition from the womb to the world. Stronger contractions work to push the baby out of the birth canal and then later help expel the placenta from the uterus now that it is no longer needed. Once your baby exits your womb and enters the world, the only remaining physical connection is the umbilical cord. However, the emotional connection, the strong and permanent bond between a mother and child, will endure for a lifetime.

DAY 190

Divine Direction

"By day the Lord *directs his love, at night his song is with me—a prayer to the God of my life."*

Psalm 42:8

There are days when it seems like I can't direct the next five minutes, much less see that God is directing my entire day. To say that I am simply forgetful or scattered is an understatement. When I am pregnant, those characteristics only increase. Knowing that God is always at work, moving and directing my steps, is so reassuring. Even when I try to make a move on my own, he is there to lead me again.

I still get lost, sidetracked, and distracted. I'll be following his path and somehow take my eyes off of him, focusing instead on a giant rock in my path. Instead of moving forward, going where he is leading me, I end up stalled or kicking the rock. Sometimes the delay is short, and often it is longer. Whether it is a pebble or a boulder obstructing my steps, he gently and lovingly helps my gaze return to him again. Where is your gaze today? Listen to his leading; fix your eyes on him. †

DAY 191

Use What You Have

"When I am afraid, I will trust in you. In God, whose word I praise, in God I trust; I will not be afraid. What can mortal man do to me?"

PSALM 56:3–4

In an effort to minimize the chaos in my life, my husband has me on the forefront of technology. My cell phone reminds me of every appointment; it checks my e-mail, keeps my calendar, and synchronizes with my home computer for up-to-the-minute updates. It works wonderfully and keeps me on track as long as I use it. But if I forget to enter a date in my calendar, then it's useless. If I forget to charge my cell phone, then no one can reach me. If I want to reap the benefits of the technology, then I have to use it properly.

God's Word works much the same way. If we are in the Word sporadically, then we forget what it says. If we don't pray, then we neglect to allow God to direct our steps. If we don't recharge our batteries by going to church, we run out of steam. Don't let yourself get out of touch with God during this pregnancy. All of your physical and emotional issues – fatigue, confusion, and uncertainty—can be combated with the restoration found in his Word. God gave us his Word as his instrument of communication; it's most effective when used consistently and frequently. Use the resources he has given you to help make your life better. †

Worthy Investments

"Why spend money on what is not bread, and your labor on what does not satisfy? Listen, listen to me, and eat what is good, and your soul will delight in the richest of fare."

ISAIAH 55:2

Our society places tremendous value in investments. We invest time in our careers, relationships, and hobbies. We invest money in our homes, clothing, education, and new technology. Everything we do is an exchange of some sort, whether time, money, or energy.

During pregnancy, you are making lots of good investments. You are purchasing items and equipment to ensure that your baby will be comfortable. Every time you eat healthy foods or follow your doctor's recommendations, you invest in your baby's health. Of all the investments you are making, are you making an investment in him?

God desires that we have an abundant life, not just a life of drudgery. He desires for you to live a life of blessing, peace, joy, and happiness. He does not desire for you to be weighed down, heavy-hearted and in turmoil. To find and live the abundant life God has for you often means investing in him so you can better find the peace and joy he has to offer you. Invest in him today. Your return will be priceless. †

DAY 193

Needing Him

"The God who made the world and everything in it is the Lord *of heaven and earth and does not live in temples built by hands. And he is not served by human hands, as if he needed anything, because he himself gives all men life and breath and everything else. . . . 'For in him we live and move and have our being.' As some of your own poets have said, 'We are his offspring.'"*

Acts 17:24–25, 28

Funny how sometimes we get into the mindset that God needs us. Sometimes our prayer life looks more like a barter system: "Okay, God, if you give me a healthy baby, I'll be better about going to church." "If you give me the raise I want, then I'll give more to the church—okay, God? Sound like a deal?" Or, "God, if somehow you ensure my husband gets a raise so we can afford a new nursery for this baby, I'll be sure to give you the glory, and I'll be a good witness. So, just give me a chance, come on, what do you say?"

God doesn't need us to be glorified. All of creation is witness to and glorifies his name. God doesn't need us to build the church; he performs the miracles and supplies the provision so that we can participate. God made it, owns it, and inhabits all of his creation. He does not need us. Conversely, we need him.

In him, we find purpose. In him, we find the living water and bread, the life everlasting. He doesn't need us to complete him. We need him to complete us. In him we have life. †

DAY 194

All His

"In bringing many sons to glory, it was fitting that God, for whom and through whom everything exists, should make the author of their salvation perfect through suffering. Both the one who makes men holy and those who are made holy are of the same family. So Jesus is not ashamed to call them brothers."

HEBREWS 2:10–11

Weeks before I was to deliver my twins, my daughter asked me, "Mommy, once the babies come, will you be able to take us out for ice cream?" Immediately I reassured her that I would. Yes, babies are a lot of work, but Mommy would still want to spend time and enjoy her as well.

When a new baby joins a family, older siblings may have mixed feelings. How will this affect their standing with Mom and Dad? Will they still be loved? Who will play with them and meet their needs? Assuring your child ahead of time of what to expect, what will stay the same and what will be different, helps those first few weeks run more smoothly.

At first, the Israelites weren't too happy about sharing their inheritance with the Gentiles. They were the rightful heirs; they were there first. Yet just as you love each of your children individually and uniquely, God similarly loves both Jew and Gentile. We are all children of the Most High. †

DAY 195

Incorruptible Inheritance

"Praise be to the God and Father of our LORD *Jesus Christ! In his great mercy he has given us new birth into a living hope through the resurrection of Jesus Christ from the dead, and into an inheritance that can never perish, spoil or fade—kept in heaven for you. . . ."*

1 PETER 1:3–4

Despite the fact that my oldest son already has three younger siblings, he remained eager to have another baby in the house until he realized that it would impact his future inheritance, splitting the dividends five ways instead of four. The allure of a younger brother or sister no longer seemed so appealing.

As parents, we want to leave each of our children an inheritance. Hopefully through wise stewardship, we will be able to provide a secure future. More than a financial inheritance, we desire to leave them a spiritual inheritance, a lasting legacy of what it means to love Christ, to walk in his ways, and to be transformed by him.

Our heavenly Father has left us the greatest inheritance we will ever receive. Regardless of the economy, our inheritance is 100 percent safe, completely intact. It will never diminish in size or lose its ability to protect and guard us. It is reserved permanently and eternally for us in heaven. Thank God for the gift of an incorruptible inheritance. †

Who Will He Be?

"You will be with child and give birth to a son, and you are to give him the name Jesus. He will be great and will be called the Son of the Most High. The Lord *God will give him the throne of his father David, and he will reign over the house of Jacob forever; his kingdom will never end."*

Luke 1:31–33

She was a poor girl, from a lowly town. She had no great name, no famous line. She was humble and simple, engaged to marry a carpenter descended from the royal line of David. She knew God intimately, and had recently seen his hand working, allowing Elizabeth to conceive despite her advanced age. She knew God performed miracles and her heart wholly loved him.

Suddenly, an angel appeared to her from nowhere, telling her that she, most favored woman, would bear no less than the Messiah—Jesus, the one who saves, the very one her family for generations had been praying for. Of all women, she would have the honor of birthing, raising, and loving the long-awaited Messiah.

God has given you charge over a child of his as well. Whose life has God given you the honor of loving and raising? Perhaps you will raise a world leader, a doctor, a passionate pastor for Christ, or maybe a teacher, a mother, a nurse, or a missionary. Who will your child be? †

DAY 197

A Different Answer

"So Pilate asked Jesus, 'Are you the king of the Jews?' 'Yes, it is as you say,' Jesus replied."

LUKE 23:3

Mary knew her child was the Messiah. Throughout his childhood, Jesus was perfect though surrounded by imperfection. He knew the Torah, sought God, and prayed without ceasing. His mother was with him when he performed his first miracle, changing the water into wine at the wedding. With each passing year, she must have wondered, when, Jesus, when? When will you reveal to the world who you are?

How differently things turned out from what she must have imagined. During her pregnancy with the Christ child, did she dream of a mighty king leading royal armies? When did she realize that the salvation he brought was not from the Romans, but from sin? When did she realize that their prayer for a Messiah had been answered, but not in the way they had imagined?

God answers prayer. He is faithful. His ways are perfect and just. He is merciful, kind, loving, wholly holy, and completely righteous. God's answers don't always look like the answer we are seeking. And often, just as through Jesus, we don't even recognize the answer he's given us. Has God been answering your prayer? Are you seeing the answer? †

DAY 198

Seek My Face

"My heart says of you, 'Seek his face!' Your face, Lord, *I will seek."*

Psalm 27:8

During the months of pregnancy, there is one face that you are longing to seek. You dream about it at night when you are sleeping, contemplating those first moments of holding your baby. Countless minutes are spent daydreaming about the little face, what features it will have, how much hair it will have, who it will resemble.

As you long to see your child's face, long to see the Father's. As you yearn to bring your baby home, do you also yearn to one day be home with your heavenly Father? What does it mean to seek his face? Seek him with all you do—your actions, your thoughts, your work, your play, and your giving. His face is easy to see; it is in everything and everywhere we go. It is in the still calm waters, it is in the clouds above. His words are there, in his Word for us to find and read. Today may your heart and mind both say, "Your face, Lord, I will seek." †

DAY 199

The Sabbath

"For in six days the LORD *made the heavens and the earth, the sea, and all that is in them, but he rested on the seventh day. Therefore the* LORD *blessed the Sabbath day and made it holy."*

EXODUS 20:11

When I was growing up as a child of the South, there were blue laws prohibiting shopping on Sundays. Little by little, the laws relaxed and the stores began opening, at first just for the afternoon, then soon for the majority of the day. Though I didn't really understand the laws as a child, I did know that Sunday was set apart, a day to be spent at home or at church with family, not at the shopping mall.

God commands us to spend the Sabbath as a day of rest. Yet in this world of constant communication and commerce, with Internet, e-mail, and 24-hour stores, we may take days off, but it is rare to have a true Sabbath. What better time than pregnancy to really begin practicing the Sabbath, allowing a reprieve from work for an entire day, without turning on the computer, returning e-mails, or making phone calls. Why not begin taking one day a week to spend resting, reading the Word, and enjoying your family? Begin now to enjoy his Sabbath gift to you. †

DAY 200

Deep Breaths

"Let everything that has breath praise the LORD. *Praise the* LORD."

PSALM 150:6

Do you find yourself breathing deeply or taking deep breaths? You know the difference. Deep breaths are what you take when your two-year-old has a complete meltdown in the middle of the grocery store or when you can't reach your feet to put on your sneakers because of your bulging belly. Then there are the times that take your breath away, the moments of joy that make you want to fully inhale motherhood: when you hear the baby's heartbeat, when you are able to get a glimpse of Baby on a sonogram, or when you feel little reassuring kicks of activity in your womb. Or when your sleepy toddler curls up in your lap for a snuggle.

Each day intertwines both kinds of moments, oscillating from deep breathing to breathing deeply. Throughout pregnancy, focus on making every moment matter, breathing deeply of the blessings God has given so that you infuse your entire being with a sense of gratitude for his presence in your life. †

DAY 201

In His Rest

"The Lord *will sustain him on his sickbed and restore him from his bed of illness."*

Psalm 41:3

Bed rest is not a welcome assignment for most women. Who wants to hear that she will be spending the remaining days of her pregnancy lying in bed? You have better things to do, like finishing the baby's room, tying up loose ends at work, spending time with your husband, and getting a pedicure! Yet, if your doctor has recommended bed rest, whether full-time or modified, the best gift you can give yourself and Baby is to heed the advice.

Rather than seeing bed rest as an obstacle, see it as a stepping-stone to a healthier outcome. The challenge of bed rest is not simply keeping your body still, but also controlling your restless spirit. If you are full of angst and worry, the purpose of bed rest is not being fulfilled. Your baby needs a mother whose body and mind are at peace, which is impossible without God. But you have the ability to cast your cares on him, knowing that your prayers are being heard. Rest in his peace. †

DAY 202

Stretch Marks

"Look to the Lord *and his strength; seek his face always. Remember the wonders he has done, his miracles, and the judgments he pronounced. . . ."*

Psalm 105:4–5

They are reddish purple, punctuating your tummy and breasts, a sure sign that exponential growth has been occurring within your body. Despite the creams and endless rubbing, they just don't seem to go away. Only time will reduce the appearance of stretch marks caused by pregnancy. Though you wish you had a magic lotion to erase the marks on your body, they are a physical sign of this pregnancy.

We have emotional stretch marks as well, from those times when we walked through the valley and experienced rapid growth, leaning on God because we had to. Though the time was hard, you became a better person for it, perhaps stronger, more compassionate, or merciful because of the trial you endured. Rather than seeing your stretch marks as something you wish you could erase, see them as reminders of the amazing gift God is giving you today. Because of how you have grown both physically and emotionally today, you will be stronger tomorrow. †

DAY 203

Nerve Pain

"Make every effort to live in peace with all men and to be holy; without holiness no one will see the LORD. *See to it that no one misses the grace of God and that no bitter root grows up to cause trouble and defile many."*

HEBREWS 12:14–15

Sciatic nerve pain is a common pregnancy complaint. When a baby settles in just the right position, it can send a streak of pain shooting down his mother's leg and lower back. Aside from delivering the baby, there are few options for relieving the pain.

Emotional pain, whether caused by the death of a loved one, a job loss, or a divorce, can also be long lasting and deeply felt. Like an open wound at risk of infection, pain from an emotional trauma can breed bitterness, anger, and additional suffering. Some pain is so acute that rather than dealing with it, allowing it to hurt and heal, it is easier to put a Band-Aid over it, ignoring the issue.

Before you bring a baby into your life, look at any emotional pain you may be still harboring. Are there people in your life you need to forgive? Or is there someone to whom you owe an apology? Rather than risking the side effects of emotional pain, take time in these last weeks to heal emotionally. You'll be better for it. †

DAY 204

Rooming In

"Evening, morning and noon I cry out in distress, and he hears my voice."

PSALM 55:17

Many moms consider rooming in, sleeping with their newborn baby nearby, during those first few weeks following her birth. Having been so close to Baby during the months of pregnancy, even being a room away seems too distant. Having Baby nearby not only makes feedings easier, it maximizes the opportunity to sleep, a precious commodity in those early weeks! It also eases concerns, knowing that Baby is okay and easily accessible. Just observing the rhythmic breathing of their newborn baby brings peace of mind to many new moms.

We room in with our heavenly Father all the time. He is beside us at all times, just as a newborn rests safely within a bassinet beside her mother's bed. Isn't it comforting to know that just as you'll hear every whimper your baby makes, he, too, hears yours? †

Names, Names

"On the eighth day, when it was time to circumcise him, he was named Jesus, the name the angel had given him before he had been conceived."

LUKE 2:21

So much thought goes into a name. It's one of the first parenting decisions you'll make for your child, and one with long-lasting consequences. You probably have a few favorites picked out. Maybe you already know the one name that is perfect for your child, or maybe you'd rather wait until after you deliver, to see what your baby looks like, before you make a decision. No doubt great thought has gone into the selection, considering your family history, the origin and meaning of the name, as well as the potential for future taunting and nicknames.

Beyond your baby's birth name, pray that your child will also become a member of the family of the Most High, and that he will also take on the name of Christ, bearing the name Christian. As you pray for your child's name and life, pray that this baby would be an individual who brings glory to the name of Jesus. Pray that your child's name will be one that is lived in honor, attracting others to the goodness of his light. †

Restful Sleep

"The Lord *replied, 'My Presence will go with you, and I will give you rest.'"*

Exodus 33:14

You probably can't remember the last time you had a truly restful night's sleep, when you weren't disturbed several times in the night by a little kick, a cramped leg, or a bathroom break. Those wakings, though annoying, are helping to condition your body's sleep cycle for the disruptive months ahead. During those first few weeks, your newborn baby will need to be fed every few hours. Waking up in the night now will make the nighttime feedings easier later.

In a few months, once your baby is able to sleep for five to six hours between feedings at night, you'll be able to really rest again, the deep, good-dreaming kind of sleeping that nearly paralyzes your entire body. Can't wait, can you?

Though God's rest can't bring relief from bath room breaks and body aches, it gives you strength to make it through the day, to find the energy to continue on when you think you could collapse. His rest sustains when physical rest is unavailable. Rest in him and allow his strength to infuse your body. †

Spiritual Milk

"Like newborn babies, crave pure spiritual milk, so that by it you may grow up in your salvation, now that you have tasted that the LORD *is good."*

1 PETER 2:2–3

There are endless opinions about how modern mothers should feed their babies, whether by breast or by bottle. My mother, who had bottle-fed both my sister and me, wasn't so sure about the breast. When I started nursing my first child, I wasn't so sure either. It hurt and I felt like my baby was always hungry. I felt inadequate; how could something so natural feel so awkward? In fact, had it not been for my husband's grandmother, who helped me through my struggle, I might have given up completely.

What is your opinion? Don't let others make this decision for you. This is your baby and your life. God has made you the mother of this child and empowered you to care for him or her. Make the best choice for you and your family. Moms crave wisdom and encouragement in the early days as much as the baby craves nourishment. Surround yourself with women who will be a blessing, not a hindrance. Give yourself the Word, spiritual milk for your hungry soul. †

Showers, Showers

"For if, by the trespass of the one man, death reigned through that one man, how much more will those who receive God's abundant provision of grace and of the gift of righteousness reign in life through the one man, Jesus Christ."

ROMANS 5:17

Picking out and registering for a car seat, layette, pacifiers, and a baby monitor is one of the most fun parts of pregnancy. Opening these gifts at a baby shower is even more fun. In a few hours you walk away blessed by the presence of friends and family who have showered you with love and gifts for Baby. Take pictures, listen to stories from others, and enjoy this special occasion in your life where your pregnancy is the main event.

You would never walk away from one of these special gifts or leave it unopened. God has given you a free gift too. God's gift of salvation through Jesus is accessible to everyone; all it requires is that the person accept it, believe in it, and receive it by faith.

A lot of people walk away from the gift. Others pick it up, study it, and put it down again, rejecting his gift. Then there are those who open it, accept it, and continue to share it with the rest of the world. Have you accepted God's gift to you? †

DAY 209

Just Being There

"For the LORD *your God is a merciful God; he will not abandon or destroy you or forget the covenant with your forefathers, which he confirmed to them by oath."*

DEUTERONOMY 4:31

Right now your baby is completely dependent on you for survival. As a child you needed your parents for everything, from applying a Band-Aid to handling a disagreement on the playground. The older you got, you probably pulled away, learning to handle obstacles and challenges on your own. Now as an adult, you know your parents hold you in their heart and are always there for you.*

Even if your earthly parents weren't there for you or no longer are, your heavenly Father is always there. He will always have the right words to say, always give you the best advice. Some days all you need is the knowledge that he is there. Other times, in the midst of struggles and hurt, you need more and you cry out to him, pleading and praying. He hears you, calms you, and restores your broken heart. He will never abandon you, he will never forsake you, he will never lie to you or become temporarily out of service. He is your eternal, righteous, loving, forgiving, and merciful father. And he is there for you. †

Living Happy

"And we know that in all things God works for the good of those who love him, who have been called according to his purpose."

ROMANS 8:28

As women, we spend a lot of time discussing our feelings with other women, our friends, mothers, and sisters. During pregnancy, feelings are especially tumultuous, ranging from elation to worry in just minutes. Feelings just happen; we can't help it if one moment we feel happy or sad, loving or unloved, angry or compassionate. Feelings come over us in waves, unexpectedly, and completely take over our state of mind. Though we can't always change how we feel, we choose how we handle those feelings.

We can change what we do with negative feelings in our life. God has given us a toolbox full of ways to help us through the feelings of despair. He has given us the Word to speak encouragement and provide examples of godly character. He has given us the Holy Spirit to indwell us, giving guidance and comfort. He has given us his Son, an everlasting and eternal hope, offering redemption from sin. Living happily every day comes from utilizing these tools and living a life in him. †

DAY 211

A Reward

"Sons are a heritage from the LORD, *children a reward from him."*
PSALM 127:3

By the end of my pregnancies, I loathed my maternity clothes. I had worn them over and over and each time I put them on, they fit worse than they did the time before. In the last days I felt like I needed a crane to get myself off the couch, and would hold my hands behind my back, helping support the load in front. Feeling physically tired, impatient, and ready to deliver, I didn't exactly feel like I was carrying around God's reward to me. I felt instead like a human barn and wasn't sure that I could do it another day.

Yet, I did. And I got bigger. Yet God sustained me and reminded me that what I was carrying was his reward, the sweetest reward. As soon as I delivered each of my children, though I had loved them passionately in the womb, I fell deeply in love and awe with each of them. Soon you'll be holding your reward. Focus on the joy of the reward to come. †

DAY 212

Live as I Do

"I have been reminded of your sincere faith, which first lived in your grandmother Lois and in your mother Eunice and, I am persuaded, now lives in you also."

2 TIMOTHY 1:5

Children are observers. They go through life and soak up like a sponge the world around them, including words they may or may not listen to and actions they may or may not emulate. As a parent, living a life worth mirroring is hard. Attending church as a family or sending your child to a school that enforces Christian values can help you in the quest to teach your child spiritual truths. Yet, ultimately the responsibility for raising your child in the way he should go lies squarely with Mom and Dad.

Teaching your child is a daily, ongoing, day-by-day experience. It begins as you wake up in the morning, and it ends as you pray with them at bedtime. They hear you say "I'm sorry" when you've made mistakes; they see you extend grace and mercy to others. When they see you love the unlovable or forgive the unforgivable, they will hopefully do the same one day. Model a life of living for God so that one day they will live as you have done, not as you have said. †

DAY 213

A Wise Steward

"His master replied, 'Well done, good and faithful servant! You have been faithful with a few things; I will put you in charge of many things. Come and share your master's happiness!'"

MATTHEW 25:21

The last few weeks have brought new meaning to the value of a minute. Each passing day, while bringing you closer to the birth, is also a day lost in preparation. There are so many details to think about, from the hospital bag to who will feed the dog while you're away to finishing up loose ends at the office. Being a wise steward of your time and resources during these last days is especially important.

God calls us to be wise stewards of all the gifts he has given us. He expects you to use your talents and abilities for his glory. He expects you to use your money and resources wisely and appropriately. He expects you to budget and balance your time among the demands of work, play, and rest. Before bringing a baby home, pregnancy allows you the opportunity to make a plan for time management later. Begin to think about how you will manage your time when the baby comes later. Good stewardship begins in good planning and preparation. †

Walking Weary

"I can do everything through him who gives me strength."
PHILIPPIANS 4:13

Toward the end of pregnancy, life seems to pass at an unbelievably slow pace, but at the same time with remarkable speed. Though the last months have passed quickly, today may feel insurmountable as you wonder how you'll make it through. In this minute you feel tired, sore, stretched, hungry, and full all at the same time. Will the day of delivery ever come?

You will get there. Live in this moment, live in his strength, not looking too far to the future and not looking at how hard it may be to get there. Instead, look at how far you've come and how much shorter the path ahead is. Remember when you waited and wondered if you were having a baby or not? His hand has crafted the miracle within you, he has protected you, and he won't stop watching over you now. Throughout this pregnancy, God has been with you. Soon you will be mothering this child. His strength will carry you. †

Without Words

"Wives, in the same way be submissive to your husbands so that, if any of them do not believe the word, they may be won over without words by the behavior of their wives, when they see the purity and reverence of your lives."

1 PETER 3:1–2

You can't make someone fall in love with you. The heart cannot always choose who it falls in love with. There is no button you can press that will control feelings, turning them on or off. Jacob, whose heart deeply loved Rachel, was first married to her sister, Leah. Leah tried to make Jacob love her, bore sons when Rachel could not, and yet it was not enough. Jacob's heart belonged to Rachel. Because love is so powerful and all consuming, often a believer finds herself married to someone who does not share her faith, hoping and praying that one day he will.

In such situations, the Word gives specific instructions. Persistent nagging is not effective in reaching the unbeliever; it does little to demonstrate the love of God. Instead, a quiet and gentle spirit, showing love through actions and acceptance, is far more fruitful. Instead of nagging and urging your husband to the church, let your love lead your husband to the cross. †

DAY 216

A New Intimacy

"His mouth is sweetness itself; he is altogether lovely. This is my lover, this my friend. . . ."

Song of Songs 5:16

Maybe it's the sheer exhaustion, the swollen feet, or the stretch marks, or perhaps it's just the enormous belly, but most moms just don't feel like their husband's sexy bride in the last weeks of pregnancy. Most women at this stage are just not eager to share intimate moments with their husband. Perhaps your sheer size is getting in the way, or maybe your doctor instructed you to abstain from marital intimacy. Whether you're feeling unsexy or are medically restricted, the frequency of intimacy is probably decreasing substantially. Yet, reconnecting as a couple is vital for a marriage in every season.

So how can you find a way to reconnect when you may not even be able to wrap your arms around him? How about a foot massage or a quiet dinner alone? Perhaps enjoying a concert, a movie, or just a quiet night at home with some soft music and conversation would be just the ticket. Initiate intimacy in new ways. Make it a point to reconnect with your husband soon. †

Loving Him

"Now go out and encourage your men. I swear by the LORD *that if you don't go out, not a man will be left with you by nightfall. . . ."*

2 SAMUEL 19:7

With all of the pregnancy preparations, expectant mommies often forget about the one who used to be their center of attention. With your words and actions, remind your husband how much you admire him, how thankful you are for him, how much you love him, and how glad you are that this baby will have him for a father. When was the last time you told him how you admire and respect him? Tell him what you think. What method you use isn't important; what matters is that you tell him. Say it out loud, perhaps while praying before a meal, or lean over and give him a kiss on the cheek and whisper something in his ear. Or tell him in writing. Hide a little love note in his briefcase or stick a Post-it note on the bathroom mirror.

Your husband yearns to hear those words of encouragement from the one person who means the most to him: you. Your words, your affirmation of your love for him, will enable him to be a better husband and father. What if you don't feel those things? Pray for those feelings to return. Ask God to show you the best in your husband, not to focus on where he is falling short. †

DAY 218

Take a Break

"After he had dismissed them, he went up on a mountainside by himself to pray. When evening came, he was there alone . . ."

MATTHEW 14:23

My ultimate indulgence is a day at the spa. Nothing relaxes me quite like the feeling of a cool cucumber towel on my eyes as I sit in the dry sauna. Basking in the Jacuzzi, listening to the musical sounds of a rain forest waterfall, the stress and tension literally melt away.

Take some time to give yourself a break. Your body has been working overtime to grow this baby, on top of your responsibilities to your job, your husband, and your home and family. Schedule a prenatal massage or treat yourself to a movie. Set aside an hour and curl up with a cup of tea and a good book. Do something that is just for you where no one else but God is invited.

As busy as Jesus was, he withdrew regularly to take little breaks. In those moments, he communed in prayer with God, allowing him to rejuvenate his soul. Use your break from the regular routine to talk to God. As you still your body from your activities, allow God to fill your quiet mind. †

DAY 219

Baby Spying

"Be dressed ready for service and keep your lamps burning, like men waiting for their master to return from a wedding banquet, so that when he comes and knocks they can immediately open the door for him."

LUKE 12:35–36

My favorite part of my prenatal checkups was what I would do after I left the doctor's office, when I'd stop by the maternity ward and visit the newborn babies. I loved seeing the grandparents share their joy, excitedly pointing out their grandchild to onlookers. I loved seeing the dads with their video cameras, recording as their tiny treasure was weighed, washed, and measured. I would leave so eager to hold my own little baby, excited to have our moment of joy, anticipating the joy to come.

God also calls us to have eager anticipation for him. Just as we can't wait for the arrival of Baby, we too should be eagerly seeking him, excited about the church service before we get there, and looking forward to an opportunity to spend time alone with him in prayer. Our hearts should be eagerly anticipating his return, having a heart ready for him when the day comes. †

DAY 220

Clock Watching

"My times are in your hands. . . ."

PSALM 31:15

How many times have you stared at your calendar, wondering which box contains the magic number, counting down to see how much longer until the day of delivery? Maybe you keep a little tally chart where you record the passing days of your pregnancy or even a countdown clock on your computer to keep you updated every time you log on. The clock moves much slower when your eyes are fixed on it. It seemingly takes forever for five minutes to pass when your gaze is on the steady movements of the second hand revolving around the clock. Instead, focus on some productive activities. These next few weeks are a great time to prepare some casseroles and freezer meals to keep on hand for easy meals after the baby's born. Or get organized by cleaning out a closet that needs tidying, making room for baby items. Take your eyes off the clock and get busy, and the time will start to fly. †

DAY 221

Defeating Boredom

"How the gold has lost its luster, the fine gold become dull! The sacred gems are scattered at the head of every street."

LAMENTATIONS 4:1

Do you feel like you are in a rut? You wake up, put on the same maternity clothes, eat the same foods, and do the same things over and over? Meanwhile, the time passes ever so slowly and you are sure that you will remain eternally pregnant.

Change up the routine. While you still can, wake up early one morning and enjoy a sunrise walk. Or try a new and different restaurant for dinner, ordering something you probably wouldn't normally select.

After dinner, have you become a couch potato, joining your husband in front of the TV until it is time for bed? Turn off the television and try reading a book together out loud, maybe a childhood favorite that you can share with your child in utero. Go to a local pond or lake and try fishing, or do something touristy in your town that you've always wanted to try. Make these last days a time to be treasured, not ones of boredom. You'll build memories to be held on to for a lifetime. †

DAY 222

The Home

"Then little children were brought to Jesus for him to place his hands on them and pray for them. . . ."

MATTHEW 19:13

You can probably visualize how different your home will look in a few weeks. Rather than a coffee table covered with magazines and decorative candles, you will have an array of receiving blankets, pacifiers, and bottles. Picture a blanket spread on the floor, with a play gym hanging overhead, baby laying underneath and gazing upward. Nearly every room will be impacted, from the highchair in the kitchen to the baby swing in the den. Everywhere there will be evidence that a baby lives in your home.

Pray over each room of your home, from the perimeter walls to the front door. Pray that within those walls, the name of Jesus would be glorified. In the bedrooms, pray that each room would be a restful sanctuary and safe haven. In the kitchen, pray that the food that is prepared would nourish your bodies and that meals would be a time of family fellowship. Bathe your home in prayer before you bring your baby home. †

DAY 223

The Grandparents

"Children's children are a crown to the aged, and parents are the pride of their children."

PROVERBS 17:6

Grandparents have the opportunity to come into a child's life as often or as little as they choose. I was fortunate enough to have grandparents who loved spending time with me, playing a game of cards, taking my sister and me to our numerous dance or piano lessons, or just enjoying an after-school snack. My grandparents gave us a most precious gift, week after week, throughout my whole life. Their gift of time was more precious and valuable, more life changing, than any monetary gift they could have given.

What kind of grandparents will your child have? Pray for the grandparents who will play a role in your child's life. Pray that they will desire to have a relationship and will invest in them with their words, prayers, and actions. Pray for the grandparents to have lives of good health and energy to keep up with a growing child. Pray that they would be a source of spiritual inheritance, leaving a legacy that transcends time as the values they impart carry from one generation to the next. †

Friendships

"Jonathan said to David, 'Go in peace, for we have sworn friendship with each other in the name of the LORD, *saying, "The* LORD *is witness between you and me, and between your descendants and my descendants forever.' . . ."*

1 SAMUEL 20:42

It may seem foolish to pray for future events when you haven't yet laid eyes on your baby. Why pray about the future when there is enough to pray about today? But God's guidance can never be sought too early or too often. Perhaps you have already prayed for your child's life, for health or safety, a seeking spirit, or even a future spouse. But have you considered praying for the friendships your child will have one day?

Just as Jesus had a circle of friends beyond his family, so will your child want companionship. It may seem like a long time away, but babies grow up very quickly. Praying for the right people in your child's life can begin now. Pray that those who are closest to your child will have a heart for Jesus, that they will be loyal friends who bring out the best characteristics in your child rather than the worst. †

Sweet Siblings

"Fathers, do not embitter your children, or they will become discouraged."

COLOSSIANS 3:21

Siblings bring a whole new dimension to the family. Getting used to a new normal, a new routine, requires everyone to make adjustments—Mom, Dad, and any older siblings. Yet, after the bumps and kinks have been worked out, what you have is a family, knit together by love and support.

In these precious weeks, as your older children are excitedly seeing the baby grow in your belly, make them a focus of your prayers. Pray that they will have full confidence in your love for them, so that if a sibling excels, they feel excitement and not jealousy. Pray that they will learn to encourage one another, feeling united as a team. Pray that you will love each one individually, not showing partiality or favoritism that sows seeds of envy and bitterness among your children. Pray that they will be better individuals because of their relationship with each other, more compassionate and sympathetic toward others, and the experience will cause them to draw closer to the image of Christ. †

Praying for Provision

"He who pursues righteousness and love finds life, prosperity and honor."

PROVERBS 21:21

Babies are expensive, even before they ever arrive. The burden of provision is one that probably weighs heavily on your husband's heart even if he is providing abundantly. Taking on the responsibility of providing for a new life, in addition to the responsibilities he already carries, can cause even the most confident man to question the future. As your husband begins to juggle the joys and responsibility of family life, encourage him with your words and prayers.

Regardless of your financial contributions, you can support your family with prayer. Thank God for the provision and blessings he has already given you, realizing how fully he has been at work in your life. Don't be afraid to name your requests for the future. Whether your financial goals are establishing a college fund, moving into a bigger house, or saving for retirement, pray for the resources, wisdom, and stewardship to help you achieve your goals. God is our ultimate provider. All we have, and all we will have, comes from him alone. †

DAY 227

On Guard

"Guard my life, for I am devoted to you. You are my God; save your servant who trusts in you."

PSALM 86:2

One of the hardest parts of parenting has been learning that I am not in control. There are spaces of the day over which I seemingly have control, like when I decide what is for dinner or what is allowed on the television, or when I direct how my children spend their time. Yet, the older my children get, the more I realize that those moments I have with them are for the purpose of preparing them for when they are not with me. They will need to know how to make wise choices about how and with whom they spend their time. Within my home, I can control what reaches their eyes and ears, but eventually I must rely on them to make good decisions.

Ultimately, all I can do is pray for them. Now is the time for you to start taking control of your prayer power. Pray for protection for your baby in the womb, during delivery, and in every moment of his life. Pray for protection from evil seen and not seen. †

Praying for Passion

"O daughters of Jerusalem, I charge you—if you find my lover, what will you tell him? Tell him I am faint with love."

SONG OF SONGS 5:8

Though you may feel passionately in love with your spouse, there may not be a lot of passion in the bedroom at this point in pregnancy. But if you and your husband have been blessed enough to share a deep, passionate love, you know that it will return. Pray for God to reveal new ways that your love can grow.

If your marriage has never known such passion, it can still be a focus of prayer. Perhaps you had passion in courtship or the early years but the weight of daily living has robbed your marriage of the passion you once knew. Pray for God to ignite your spirit with a new love. Pray for him to help show you ways to develop passion, whether it is in finding a common thread in the sharing of interests and desires or finding a new way to love. God desires your marriage to be a source of great joy to you. Pray that you have a marriage that is deep and fulfilling for you both. †

DAY 229

Working Moms

"So whether you eat or drink or whatever you do, do it all for the glory of God."

1 CORINTHIANS 10:31

When you become a mother, you take on the most important job title of your life. While some women make motherhood their sole job description for a period of time and others choose to balance a career with the work of motherhood, all moms are working mothers. As you make the difficult decisions about staying at home, working, child care, and more, ask God to lead you in your preparations.

God chooses to use and work through each of us differently. He might place one woman in a career, and his will is to continue her path in that job while she raises her children. God places other women at home, giving them this season of mothering away from the marketplace. Wherever you feel God is directing you, check that you are doing it for God's will and not your own. A woman can choose to stay at home for the wrong reasons just as a woman can choose to continue working for the wrong motive. Search your heart, pray, and ask God to show you where you belong. †

DAY 230

HELP!

"May the Lord *answer you when you are in distress; may the name of the God of Jacob protect you. May he send you help from the sanctuary and grant you support from Zion."*

Psalm 20:1–3

The reason I had any semblance of sanity during my twins' first year was due to the help of my housekeeper. Six days a week my house resembled a day camp designed for children aged five and under, but one day a week it had order. The weekly reprieve meant my clothes were washed and ironed; my floors were mopped and vacuumed; my toilets, bathtubs, and showers were clean. The responsibility of caring for four little lives, a husband, and a home were all I could take. Having her come behind me once a week, doing the big tasks I could not, was literally a lifesaver.

What kind of help will you need once the baby arrives? Will you need domestic help? Help with meals? Help with picking up other children? As these weeks pass, begin to line up those who will help you with the weeks ahead, praying and asking God to partner you with the perfect complementary help for your family. †

DAY 231

Bag Packing

"Your word is a lamp to my feet and a light for my path."

PSALM 119:105

In the next few weeks you will probably want to have your hospital bag packed and ready, even if you are scheduled for a C-section or induction of labor. Babies and bodies don't always cooperate with calendars, and having the bag ready and accessible will reduce your stress if your labor happens earlier than expected.

What should you pack? Soothing music, an outfit for baby, and one for you, too. However, don't pack your favorite prepregnancy jeans and T-shirt. It could take several weeks for your body to return to normal, and you may find it most comfortable to leave the hospital in the clothes you wore in. Bring along some comfort items, like lotion, and comfortable socks, nursing bras, lip balm, some soothing music, a camera, and most importantly, your Bible.

In his Word, God has packed everything we need to get us through each day. We can find a dose of encouragement, a word of wisdom, healing for hurting hearts. What has he packed in the Bible just for you today? †

DAY 232

Baby Needs

"May he strengthen your hearts so that you will be blameless and holy in the presence of our God and Father when our LORD *Jesus comes with all his holy ones."*

1 THESSALONIANS 3:13

Though Baby arrives at the hospital with everything she needs within the safe confines of mom's womb, the journey home requires a few more supplies. Your baby will need clothes, blankets, diapers and wipes, perhaps bottles or a pacifier, and a bag to contain it all. Most importantly, she'll have to ride home in an approved infant car seat, so check the requirements for your state. As you begin preparing for the journey to the hospital, prepare as well for your departure both from the hospital and once you arrive home. Do you have any preparation left for the baby's needs at home?

Isn't it nice that God is prepared for us at all times? We don't have to prepare to seek him, he is always there. We don't have to prepare our eternal home; it has been prepared for us. We only have to prepare our hearts, being willing always to walk in his will, seeking him, wanting him. †

DAY 233

Setting Expectations

"But the wisdom that comes from heaven is first of all pure; then peace-loving, considerate, submissive, full of mercy and good fruit, impartial and sincere."

JAMES 3:17

Many a new mom experiences disappointment and emotional upheaval when her husband doesn't meet her expectations during childbirth, delivery, and the postpartum period. Maybe she thought he'd say or do something different while she was in labor or expected him to clean up the house before she returned from the hospital. A little bit of honest communication in advance of the event can help diffuse the hurt feelings exacerbated by the physical and hormonal upheaval that follows childbirth.

God sets expectations for us also. He expects us to live a life of righteousness in response to his love for us. He expects us to be a light, a shining illumination to those lost in this dark world. Just as your husband may fall short in what you expect from him, we too fall short of what we have been asked. Just as God gives you grace every time and in every way we don't measure up, be full of grace in this time to your husband, realizing that he loves you and is trying to do his best. †

The Delivery Room

"In the same way, I tell you, there is rejoicing in the presence of the angels of God over one sinner who repents."

LUKE 15:10

Whether you deliver in a hospital, at home, or in a birthing center, you will decide who will be present with you when your baby is born. Perhaps you want to celebrate this intimate moment alone with your husband, or desire the female companionship of your mother, mother-in-law, sister, or close friend. If you have a doula attending the birth, she will be present, acting as your advocate and ensuring your requests are honored.

Where were you when you passed from death to life? What was your delivery room of salvation? Did you discover Jesus in a church, with a friend, or in a motel room? Whether you gave your heart to Jesus at a camp as a youth or over a Bible study as an adult, you were delivered, redeemed, and passed from a life of hopelessness to one of hope. †

DAY 235

Visitation Hours

"When it was time for Elizabeth to have her baby, she gave birth to a son. Her neighbors and relatives heard that the LORD *had shown her great mercy, and they shared her joy."*

LUKE 1:57–58

Each of my four children had a unique and different delivery. Following each birth, I was able to share the joyous miracle with the friends and family who gathered around us; the moments are some of my most treasured memories of life. When my sister gave birth, she preferred to have a more private delivery, wanting to share the first few days quietly with her husband and child and waiting to receive guests until after she returned home.

God made every woman different, and the way each mother wants to experience her delivery is different. Have you thought about your preferences? If you would prefer to have time to yourself before you share your baby with the world, lovingly and gently tell your loved ones what your plans are, to reduce hurt feelings later. Setting expectations early and clearly helps your husband and close family members make this time everything you desire. †

DAY 236

Hospital Beds

"Here I am! I stand at the door and knock. If anyone hears my voice and opens the door, I will come in and eat with him, and he with me."

REVELATION 3:20

After I delivered my first child, my husband spent the night cramped on a cot the nurse brought to my hospital room. As if the cot wasn't uncomfortable enough for his tall frame, I kept waking him up to marvel about the miracle of our baby. With our other babies, he chose to spend the nights at home with our older children, bringing them to the hospital after the deliveries. Though it may seem like a great idea to have your spouse sleep over with you, consider that it will be a great benefit to have at least one set of rested eyes for the nights ahead.

From the rushed delivery room where baby's arrival is anxiously anticipated to the still of the night when you hold her alone, just the two of you for the first time, God will be there through it all. He will not leave you when you are scared, and he will celebrate with you in the joy and relief. Anticipate him, expect him, and include him in your delivery experience. †

DAY 237

Baby Watch

"Therefore keep watch, because you do not know on what day your LORD *will come."*

MATTHEW 24:42

You've probably memorized all of the signs and symptoms of labor by now.

Sisters and girlfriends have shared their stories and theories; contractions, bloody show, lightening, ruptured membranes. Often the signs are more subtle, evolving slowly day by day, without flashy show or drama, but a simple drawing near. Whether your labor story will be as dramatic as your water breaking in a restaurant or as expected as a scheduled C-section, you are watching, readying yourself for the time.

God also has told us signs to look for so we are ready for Christ's return. It is easy to look at today's events as clear signs that he is coming soon. Yet, the Word says we should not concern ourselves over the day or time, just that we should be ready whenever it comes. We should be on guard, watching, waiting, seeing him move in our life and knowing that he will return. Are you on watch for him? †

DAY 238

Pain Relief

"When my spirit grows faint within me, it is you who know my way. . . ."

Psalm 142:3

I thought I would give natural childbirth a try, but I planned to request an epidural should the pain become too intense. Had I realized I was actually in labor, an epidural may have been an option. Instead I mistook my labor pains for an upset stomach and kept leaving the dinner table to dash to the restroom. It wasn't until my husband and I returned home that we realized it was probably labor. By the time we arrived at the hospital, it was time to deliver. I had a natural birth after all.

Life doesn't always go according to our plan. When trials hit or things take an unexpected turn, faith keeps us on course. Even when the path is difficult to see, or when we feel unsure of whether to go right or left, as long as our steps are steadied in him, we will end exactly where he has planned. †

DAY 239

Blink of an Eye

"But blessed is the man who trusts in the Lord, *whose confidence is in him."*

Jeremiah 17:7

The passing of time during pregnancy is a paradox. Never has time moved so slowly yet so quickly at the same time. Here you stand at the door of the last month of the last trimester. You can either fixate your thoughts on how uncomfortable you feel, how much weight you've gained, and how you can't sleep, or you can choose to cherish these last days.

Next month, it won't be quite as easy to enjoy a quiet meal in a restaurant with your husband. Rather than rereading pregnancy books and surfing baby Web sites, spend the evening together, taking a walk or watching a movie. You have the choice to cherish or to complain; how you spend these last days is your decision.

Throughout life we also have the same decision. No season of life is without some blemishes. God asks us to cherish the blessings he has given us whether we are in a season of plenty or in need. You have been blessed. †

Who Am I?

"'But what about you?' he asked. 'Who do you say I am?' Simon Peter answered, 'You are the Christ, the Son of the living God.'"

MATTHEW 16:15–16

What are you having? When are you due? How much longer do you have? Are you having a C-section? What is the baby's name? Where will you deliver? Sound familiar? You've been barraged with questions throughout this pregnancy, and by now you may have some answers.

At some point in your life you may also be asked another question: "Who is Jesus?" or "Are you a Christian?" or "What religion are you?" It is much like when Jesus asked Peter, "Who do you say I am?" Do you have an answer? When given the chance to share about Jesus, what do you say? Peter answered, "You are the Christ," meaning Messiah, the one who saves. Don't miss an opportunity to tell others about the One who saves; have an answer ready. †

DAY 241

Special Presents

"If you, then, though you are evil, know how to give good gifts to your children, how much more will your Father in heaven give good gifts to those who ask him!"

MATTHEW 7:11

My daughter was thrilled with her new pink purse; it made her feel like a beautiful movie star instead of the three-year-old big sister of newborn twin brothers. She was excited about those little bundles in the corner, oh yeah, those babies, but the thing she was really excited about was the gifts from well-meaning visitors who were kind enough to include her and her older brother with a small token of remembrance.

Having a special present or prize for your child is a way of including him or her in the birth of your new baby and may help minimize resentment about the attention that is now being directed to a little seven-pound bundle rather than him or her.

Throughout each day, God gives us special, small gifts reminding us of his presence. Sometimes it is a convenient parking space or a beautiful sunrise only his hands could paint or a kind word of encouragement from a friend. Recognize the little gifts in your life and relish the love he has lavished on you. †

DAY 242

Time to Prune

"I am the true vine, and my Father is the gardener. He cuts off every branch in me that bears no fruit, while every branch that does bear fruit he prunes so that it will be even more fruitful."

John 15:1–2

Pruning isn't exactly my favorite way to spend an afternoon. Sweating in the hot sun helping my husband trim back our hedges, bushes, and trees is hard work, but at the end of the day, we always stand back admiring our work and the beauty it bears. Not only does our lawn look better instantly, but there are more flowers, more fruit, and healthier plants. To keep a tree healthy and beautiful or to keep bushes from becoming overgrown and in disarray requires pruning.

The same is true when we are pruned spiritually. Because we abide in Christ, the living vine, we will all bear fruit. When we go through a period of pruning, such as a trial, disappointment, or time of waiting, the lesson isn't easy. But God says we will be even better than before because of the pruning. Because of the tribulation, we learn to lean on God in a new way or learn compassion previously unknown. Each pruning brings us a little closer to the image of Christ. †

The Right Clothes

"Suppose a man comes into your meeting wearing a gold ring and fine clothes, and a poor man in shabby clothes also comes in. If you show special attention to the man wearing fine clothes and say, 'Here's a good seat for you,' but say to the poor man, 'You stand there' or 'Sit on the floor by my feet,' have you not discriminated among yourselves and become judges with evil thoughts?"

JAMES 2:2–4

It never occurred to me to bring a nightgown from home to wear after delivery. I wore the standard-issue hospital gown instead, risking exposure every time I fed my son. It was tricky to figure out breast-feeding and simultaneously be discreet. With subsequent deliveries, I was smarter, packing not only proper nursing nightgowns, but also balms for the soreness that developed in the first few days of nursing.

Though there are "right" clothes for a pregnant and nursing mom, we don't have to have a "right" look for Christ. He sees us the same regardless of the fashion statements we make. Whether we wear clothes that are two years old or fresh off the rack, he sees us no differently. He asks that we do the same to others. We aren't to prejudge people or show favoritism to others based on their attire. Our eyes should see others as Christ sees them—the lost, the hungry, full of needs, desperately needing the touch of Christ. †

DAY 244

Him First

"Anyone who loves his father or mother more than me is not worthy of me; anyone who loves his son or daughter more than me is not worthy of me. . . ."

MATTHEW 10:37

You can truthfully say that Baby has come perilously close to holding the number one priority slot since you became pregnant. Physically it has hijacked your body, so thinking about much else is often impossible. After Baby comes, the physical and emotional demands of babies and children make it easy to keep the child in the number one slot. God wants us to love our children, to be good parents of the blessing he has given us. Yet, he doesn't want our child to replace the most important priority, him.

When God is first, our families and our relationships are in healthy alignment, enabling us to be better mothers, better wives, and better friends. Loving your child more causes problems: Marital division, hindered prayer life, a disconnected walk with God. No child is served, and, in fact, the child is dishonored, by living a life where she is more important than God. Don't let the trappings of pregnancy and babyhood push God out of place in your life. Firmly establish him as your first priority, the head of your life, marriage, and family. †

DAY 245

Pregnant Forever

"May the God of hope fill you with all joy and peace as you trust in him, so that you may overflow with hope by the power of the Holy Spirit."

Romans 15:13

It will never come. I will always be pregnant. I am going to look this way forever." Have you muttered these statements in moments of weariness and fatigue? Despite the fact that it is a medical impossibility for you to remain eternally pregnant, it feels like you might. Even though the day of delivery is only a few weeks away, it may as well be another year because of the fatigue you feel right now.

It's easy to get fatigued in other aspects of life. "My life will never get better . . ." "He will never change; it will always be this way . . ." "We will never get out of this financial stress . . ." We've spoken defeat, given up. The enemy didn't even have to expend any of his own energy; we did the work for him. We serve a God of hope, not hopelessness. Because of him, in any situation we can be filled with all joy and all peace abounding in hope. You have hope in him. †

Flavored with Love

"Do everything in love."

1 CORINTHIANS 16:14

In some situations, love just occurs naturally. You don't have to make yourself love the baby you are carrying. You just do. You can't help but love your child, stirred to a new depth of emotion and level of protectiveness that you didn't even know existed. Then there are times when love doesn't come naturally. If your words are hurtful to someone else, even if they were truthful, they were probably said without love. Love has a way of seasoning what we say and what we do. When we do something motivated by love, it is received better. Our words are listened to and accepted for their value. When we approach others with a judgmental attitude of spiritual superiority or condemnation, our words and actions will only drive the person further away from the Cross.

Before you act, pray for love. If you don't feel it, pray until you do. Let your actions be flavored with love; all else will fail. †

DAY 247

The Tears of Jesus

"Jesus wept."

JOHN 11:35

There is one place in Scripture where we see our strong Savior weep. Jesus learned that Lazarus, his dear friend, had passed. When Mary, Lazarus's sister, said to him, "LORD, if you had been here, my brother would not have died" in disappointed tears, Jesus groaned in response and was troubled. Mary, who knew he was capable of miraculous healing, assumed it was too late.

How often are we like Mary or Lazarus, wearing grave clothes though we walk in his life? Because the answer wasn't given on our timeline we believe that the answer was no. Does God just look at us, saying too, Believe, wait, you'll see the glory of God? Christ could have healed Lazarus's illness, but instead he raised him from the dead. Maybe, like Lazarus, your yes came later than expected. Perhaps you prayed for a baby and waited years before God finally allowed conception. Or perhaps you've been praying for a healing, a job, or a situation for so long with no response that you groan like Mary, "It's too late!" What are you filled with sadness over? What has weighed down your heart? God has not forgotten. You will see the glory of God. †

Childhood Commitments

"Show me your ways, O Lord, *teach me your paths; guide me in your truth and teach me, for you are God my Savior, and my hope is in you all day long."*

Psalm 25:4–5

You are about to become a mother, making one of the biggest commitments of your life. You, above all, are responsible for the physical and spiritual nurturing of your child. Nurturing happens every day, not just one hour per day or one week out of a month. It is a moment-by-moment experience. Just as you can't decide, "Today I won't be pregnant; I'll pick it back up tomorrow," the same is true with parenting. Even on the days when you are tired, weary, having a crisis at work, or sick with the flu, you will still be your child's mother.

Society gives modern parents plenty of "outs"; while computers, television, activities, and child care can be valuable tools, parents can overuse them as substitutes for parenting. Ultimately, though, the responsibility for raising this child won't rest on the church's Sunday school class, your child's school, or even your spouse. You have been given charge over your child; how will you fulfill this commitment? †

DAY 249

Longing Arms

"Now we know that if the earthly tent we live in is destroyed, we have a building from God, an eternal house in heaven, not built by human hands. Meanwhile we groan, longing to be clothed with our heavenly dwelling. . . ."

2 CORINTHIANS 5:1–2

You haven't yet laid eyes on this child, but your arms long to hold her. Though she is physically in close proximity, inches from your heart, eating what you eat, drinking what you drink, you feel a great distance between you. You feel a deep sense of longing that will be filled only by holding her in your arms.

You may have felt the same way before your own rebirth in Christ. Though he was all around you, loving you, nourishing you, keeping you safe, you felt so very far away because you had not trusted in him. The doubts and questions about your purpose in this world created a void in your soul that could be filled only by him. Just as joy will fill your soul when you finally hold the baby your arms long to hold, so the LORD was filled with joy when you decided to trust in him as he wrote your name in the Book of Life. †

DAY 250

No Sweeter Smell

". . . When Isaac caught the smell of his clothes, he blessed him and said, 'Ah, the smell of my son is like the smell of a field that the Lord *has blessed.'"*

Genesis 27:27

There is nothing quite like the smell of a newborn baby, freshly bathed and slathered in baby lotion. It will be a smell that you will sear into your memory, and every time you smell baby lotion, you will instantly be reminded of the early days of motherhood. In a few weeks, you'll be spending a lot of time holding your baby, nuzzling her close, whispering affectionate words in her ear, and telling her how much you love her. You'll check on her countless times as she sleeps, just to ensure she is still breathing, that everything is okay. Many minutes will be spent in awe, gazing in awe and admiration at your baby who is the miraculous culmination of the love between you and your husband.

God spends time gazing at, listening to, and loving us. He continually keeps guard over us, watching us in our comings and goings, as we sleep and as we are awake. You are to him the sweet fragrance of his daughter, the one he loves. †

DAY 251

A New Name

"You gave me life and showed me kindness, and in your providence watched over my spirit."

Job 10:12

If you've ever been on a playground when a child called, "Mommy!" you've seen women's heads swivel from all around the park. Are you ready to turn your head to the call of motherhood? Somehow you will be able to discern your child's cry in a sea of children, knowing instantly that it is your own. Nothing will comfort your child more than your response, the loving arms that will embrace him, the kiss that will take away the sting of the fall, or the shoulder to sob on. You are this child's mother, and even well after the child is grown and lives far away, nothing will bring comfort like the soothing words of Mom.

Of all the prayers offered up simultaneously every moment, God hears your voice when you pray to him. He knows who is asking and listens. In a sea of requests, he takes the time to hear your hurt. He is your Father. †

DAY 252

Protective Presentation

"Therefore put on the full armor of God, so that when the day of evil comes, you may be able to stand your ground, and after you have done everything, to stand."

EPHESIANS 6:13

As space in your womb becomes tight, baby's movements decrease and he may settle into a presenting position, ready for delivery. Whether head down, breech, or transverse, the positioning for childbirth is important. It helps reduce the risk of complications and caesarean birth, and diminishes stress on the baby. Likewise, when we are spiritually in the right position, we stand stronger against complications and stress.

Putting on the armor of God gives us the proper presentation to face the battles of life. Spiritual armor is described in Ephesians 6:14–18 and includes the belt of truth, the breastplate of righteousness, feet fitted with readiness, the shield of faith, the helmet of salvation, and the sword of the Spirit, which is the Word of God. Clothe yourself with this armor to prepare for the adventure ahead. †

DAY 253

Instruction Manual

"The Sovereign Lord *has given me an instructed tongue, to know the word that sustains the weary. He wakens me morning by morning, wakens my ear to listen like one being taught."*

Isaiah 50:4

As much as I knew about pregnancy, I felt pretty clueless when it came to actually having a baby. Sure I had plenty of books on my shelf, but there was no specific manual for my baby. There was no instruction book that explained why my baby was crying or what I should do to make him stop. Everything was conflicting opinion: pick him up if he cries, put him down if he cries. Wake him up, let him sleep. Feed him on demand, feed him on a schedule. How could the books know what was right for my baby; he was surely different than any other baby out there. Individual babies have individual needs. How was I supposed to discern what was right for my baby?

Fortunately, God gives mothers instinct and direction. He gives us support and encouragement from the mothers, grandmothers, sisters, and girlfriends in our lives, and guidance from doctors, midwives, doulas, and lactation consultants. He also gives us his Word, an instruction manual for all aspects of life. †

A Pure Love

"Can a mother forget the baby at her breast and have no compassion on the child she has borne? . . ."

ISAIAH 49:15

When the Bible gives a word picture of how God loves each of us, it is no mistake that he uses a description of a mother and her baby. The nursing mother provides the ultimate lifeline for baby, providing sustenance all day long. She loves her child with a pure love, one that is not tainted with disappointment. The child has not yet gotten old enough to disobey, talk back, or have an attitude. Her love is a clean slate for a life full of possibility and hope. The love is protective, not wanting a hair on the baby's head to be harmed.

As strong as a nursing mother's love is for her baby, God loves you even more. He sees you as his own. He sees you not for what you have done wrong in your life, but with the potential you have to succeed. He sees you as his perfect creation, the one he loves so much that he sent Jesus to die so that he would never have to be separated from you. †

DAY 255

Power of Touch

"Jesus reached out his hand and touched the man. 'I am willing,' he said. 'Be clean!' Immediately he was cured of his leprosy."

MATTHEW 8:3

Babies thrive on touch. Modern medicine points to the power of touch as a source of increased growth and diminished pain. Babies who are touched and massaged regularly have a decrease in autoimmune problems and are more alert. Just the touch of Mom, Dad, a nurse, or a doctor can produce so many amazing results.

We also require touch. Like in the way your husband can hold you and ease your pain without ever saying a word. Or a hug from a friend, a pat on the hand that is a reassuring signal of her support. Touch conveys care, compassion, and love.

As much as we thrive from the touch of others, there is one touch we all require; the touch of Jesus. He is our healer, touching us in ways we can't comprehend. He is our redeemer, touching us with salvation. As believers in Christ we are compelled to share it with others, a touch that delivers a thriving life. †

DAY 256

Passing Time

"'Martha, Martha,' the Lord *answered, 'you are worried and upset about many things, but only one thing is needed. Mary has chosen what is better, and it will not be taken away from her.'"*

Luke 10:41–42

I wanted to stay busy. I thought the busier I stayed, the more quickly the days would pass. If the days passed quickly, then I would be holding my baby sooner. It's easy to take on the role of Martha in life. We get busy running errands, working out, parenting kids, volunteering, pursuing careers. We're even busy in our leisure time, playing sports and scheduling our hobbies. In fact we are so busy sometimes that the days pass so quickly from one to the next, indistinguishable, a blur, so that we forget to pause, breathe, enjoy the exact moment we are in right now.

Mary wasn't ignoring the things that needed to be done. Yet the Lord himself commended her choice to linger at the feet of Jesus, drinking in his words. In these last days, don't busy yourself so much that you overlook these precious moments. Slow down, savor each moment, and really live in the moment. The next one will come all too soon. For now, enjoy what is better. †

Tricks of the Trade

"For great is your love, higher than the heavens; your faithfulness reaches to the skies."

PSALM 108:4

My sister drank castor oil, felt horrible, and was still pregnant. My best friend walked three miles every morning, which was great exercise but did little to facilitate her dilation. I ate Mexican food and just got heartburn. We've all heard the "tricks of the trade," things that may entice the body into labor. Sex, spicy foods, raspberry tea, pineapples, and herbs are all supposed to help speed things along. For those that claim success with these measures, more often than not, they didn't actually prompt the onset of labor but just happened to correspond with the body's natural timing.

Just as we can't "do" anything that makes God love us any more or less, there isn't much you can do that will entice your body into labor. Both just happen. Instead of trying so hard to force the inevitable, just live knowing the time will come. †

DAY 258

Love Letters

". . . For out of the overflow of his heart his mouth speaks."

Luke 6:45

Is your heart overflowing with emotion toward your baby, so much so that you can't seem to stop thinking or talking about her? There is so much to tell her and so much you want her to know. You've probably told her how you love her and can't wait to see her. You've probably called her by her name, nicely asking her to move a bit so you could find some relief from pain or a reprieve from the restroom. Maybe you've told her about her room, her dog, her grandparents and siblings or cousins. Consider writing down these emotions and feelings in a love letter to her, a keepsake you can keep for perhaps when she is pregnant with her own child.

God has given us a love letter too. In his Word we discover who he is, why he created us, who we are in relation to him, what he is capable of, and how much he loves us. Have you read his love letter to you lately? †

DAY 259

Different Plans

"'For I know the plans I have for you,' declares the LORD, *'plans to prosper you and not to harm you, plans to give you hope and a future.'"*

JEREMIAH 29:11

Scheduled for an induction, I had planned every detail of my labor, imagining myself sucking on ice chips while meditating to music as a backdrop to our prayers. But waking up in severe pain at 5:00 A.M. two days before I was scheduled to be at the hospital was not part of the plan. My husband took on the persona of an Indy 500 driver, challenged by the thrill of rushing his wife to the hospital and beating an oncoming freight train across the railroad tracks. I wasn't sure if my heart was racing because of the labor pains or the near-death experience.

Like most of life, the reality of an event is often different from what we've envisioned. The Jews wanted a savior from Roman oppression. Instead, Christ delivered them from the oppression of sin. The king of kings should not have been born in a dirty stable, but amidst the finest royalty and riches. Often his will, his perfect plan, doesn't resemble our intentions. Be willing to walk according to his plan, and don't be disappointed by a turn of events. †

DAY 260

False Labor

"What good is it, my brothers, if a man claims to have faith but has no deeds? Can such faith save him? . . . In the same way, faith by itself, if it is not accompanied by action, is dead."

JAMES 2:14, 17

In the last weeks I was certain I was in labor no less than four times a day. I would notice my Braxton Hicks contractions increasing and think "This is it!" An hour would pass and so would the contractions. What differentiates false labor from real labor is that the contractions produce no progression, neither dilating nor effacing the cervix. Real labor—regular, consistent contractions that increase in number and strength—usually has other hallmarks too, such as the bloody show or broken water. It is hard to differentiate between false and real labor, especially when you're eager and anxious.

What differentiates a church attendee from a Christ believer? Like Braxton Hicks and true labor contractions, they often look the same: they show up every Sunday, sing the same songs, and even contribute to the church family. Yet, a true believer has progression, allowing God to work on her heart through the leading of the Holy Spirit. True believers have admitted their need for Christ. A Christ believer doesn't just put in an appearance, but has been transformed by the presence of Christ in her life. †

A Circumcised Heart

d the God of Jews only? Is he not the God of Gentiles es, of Gentiles too, since there is only one God, who will the circumcised by faith and the uncircumcised through ame faith."

ROMANS 3:29–30

he thought of my little boy babies being circumcised caused me to cringe. I didn't want to think about my sweet little darlings feeling discomfort so soon after delivery. My only consolation was the fact that they would not remember the event. Within minutes of each circumcision, I was able to comfort them.

Circumcision was performed to distinguish and separate the Jewish people from the rest of the world. As circumcised males, they were set apart, made different for the purpose of God. You may be considering circumcision for medical, personal appearance or preference, or religious reasons. Whether you choose circumcision or not for your child, God calls us to be set apart and distinguishable with a circumcised heart. †

Last Meal

"And he took bread, gave thanks and broke it, and gave it to them, saying, 'This is my body given for you; do this in remembrance of me.' In the same way, after the supper he took the cup, saying, 'This cup is the new covenant in my blood, which is poured out for you.'"

LUKE 22:19–20

Will it be tonight? Do you wonder if each meal might be your last—before Baby that is? If your body isn't cooperating with your timeline, you might end up having a string of last dinners, last bedtimes, and last nights alone with your husband. Enjoy each special day as though it were the last, each baby kick as though you may never feel it again, and the swell of your tummy as though it could be gone tomorrow.

Jesus knew with certainty when he shared his last supper with the disciples, though the disciples did not. He sat among his friends and students, including the one who would soon betray him, and tried one last time to impart to them what was about to happen. He broke bread, drank wine, and asked the disciples to do this in remembrance of him. They didn't know the broken bread was a symbol of his body, or that the cup signified his blood that was about to be shed for them. †

Audible Prayers

"I pray that out of his glorious riches he may strengthen you with power through his Spirit in your inner being, so that Christ may dwell in your hearts through faith. . . ."

EPHESIANS 3:16–17

I began praying for each of my children before they were born and continue to pray for them every day. Every night my husband and I pray audibly over them. Prayer is a time for us to reconnect with God and with them, an important strand in our family's DNA.

Our bedtime prayers allow us jointly to bring our praises and requests to the throne of God, but the routine also serves a practical purpose. First, our children, at least once throughout the day, are validated. Even if we have had to discipline them earlier in the day, they hear that we love them and are proud of them. Second, it teaches them how to pray themselves. As long as we can, we will intercede in prayer for them, but it is important they learn themselves how to talk to God. How will you bring prayer into your family life? Decide in pregnancy how to integrate prayer, and when Baby is born, begin immediately to practice it. Make family prayer a lasting legacy in you. †

Nesting Now

"He who dwells in the shelter of the Most High will rest in the shadow of the Almighty."

PSALM 91:1

Despite your enormous size, you find yourself on hands and knees scrubbing the baseboards or dragging out the ladder trying to balance yourself as you clean cobwebs in the corners. Are you nesting? Most pregnant women experience this compulsion as the day of delivery draws near, madly cleaning, organizing, washing, and otherwise readying the home for the new arrival. Perhaps your body instinctively realizes it may be a while before you are able to perform such in-depth cleaning again.

Just as you are preparing your home, God goes before us, preparing not only our hearts, but others for our interactions with them. He lights our path, providing guidance even in moments when darkness consumes us or when we are unsure of which road to take. When we are living a life in partnership with him, it is impossible to go down an uncharted road, for he has gone before us, leading the way. †

DAY 265

Worth the Wait

"For in this hope we were saved. But hope that is seen is no hope at all. Who hopes for what he already has? But if we hope for what we do not yet have, we wait for it patiently."

Romans 8:24–25

I'd read that babies could safely be delivered at week 38. So what was the point of waiting? Why not just schedule an appointment, start the induction, and get the show on the road? Because waiting, as hard and tedious as it may seem, is still better. There will be less stress on baby, less medical intervention, more time for little lungs to strengthen and reflexes to develop. There is still plenty of reason to wait.

When God wants us to wait, it always serves a purpose. Waiting creates an attitude of gratitude and thanksgiving, a realization that things could be different. Waiting creates perseverance. Waiting generates compassion. Wait without grumbling, but expectantly knowing that what you have is worth the wait. †

DAY 266

When Something Goes Wrong

"The Lord *himself goes before you and will be with you; he will never leave you nor forsake you. Do not be afraid; do not be discouraged."*

Deuteronomy 31:8

We don't understand when something goes wrong. We want to have a reason or point blame. When you are going through a major trial in your life, such as receiving a bad medical report, the very core of your faith can be questioned. Because God has given us free choice, many times we find ourselves in the cross fire of consequences from others' bad choices. Though God doesn't cause sickness or birth defects, he is able to heal, restore, or show blessing even in the midst of bad circumstances, revealing his glory in the smallest details.

Unlike the unbeliever who faces these situations alone, we have hope. We have the great "I Am," who walks with us in times of uncertainty. We have the great Providence directing our steps to the medical directors, going before us in the operation rooms, pairing us with mentors, finding supporters who have walked the road before us. He does not leave us or forsake us. He is always there. †

DAY 267

So Scared

"While they were there, the time came for the baby to be born, and she gave birth to her firstborn, a son. She wrapped him in cloths and placed him in a manger, because there was no room for them in the inn."

LUKE 2:6–7

She felt the pains coming, intensifying. Was she scared as her eyes surveyed the crowded city and the roomless inns, smelling the stench in the streets? She knew she was carrying the Messiah; surely God would not have her deliver on a donkey. As the labor intensified, Joseph's pleas for help must have been desperate. Seeing their need, someone directed them to the only thing they could think of, not a clean room in the inn, but a cave used for stabling animals. Instead of medical professionals, she had only the support of her husband and, most importantly, she had her God.

You probably feel scared about childbirth, too. Despite the fact that modern birthing facilities are outfitted with the latest medical innovations, wi-fi for your laptop, comfortable couches, and an entertainment system, it doesn't change the fact that delivery is scary. You do not go into the delivery room alone. At your disposal you have what Mary had as she delivered the Messiah. You have your Father. You have God. †

In His Strength

"My hand will sustain him; surely my arm will strengthen him."
PSALM 89:21

She was enormous. And stuck. I was sure of it. I kept hearing my husband saying, "PUSH, baby, PUUSSSHHHH!" Did he think I was just relaxing, enjoying the remote-control bed? I was pushing with all of my might, screaming at the top of my lungs, and that little baby was just not going to move. Though I was sure I was depleted, God strengthened me. After a few more "good" pushes, we had a big, beautiful, healthy baby girl.

There is no denying that labor pains hurt, that there are moments when it feels like the body is not capable of doing the task before it. But God will give you the strength, the stamina, the ability to deliver your child. When you are sure you can't push another time, somehow he will enable you to. If delivering by C-section, he will be with you in the operating room. Whether you have a C-section or a vaginal birth, when you deliver the baby, you'll know everything you went through was well worth the reward. †

DAY 269

The First Days

"Let the peace of Christ rule in your hearts, since as members of one body you were called to peace. And be thankful."

COLOSSIANS 3:15

I had a pretty good idea of what to expect during pregnancy, labor, and delivery. Yet, I hadn't given much thought to what would happen after that. After carrying and birthing a baby, a woman's body still has some work to do. Hormones go into overdrive as the body switches functions from growing the baby in the womb to nourishing the baby outside the womb, producing colostrum and milk in the breasts. The body also must heal the scars of giving birth, whether an incision from a C-section or an episiotomy after vaginal delivery.

Feeling out of sync for a few weeks is completely normal. God's peace is always accessible, before and after delivery, whether you are blissfully holding your child or feeling sore and sleepy. Every day you will heal a little more. Your hormones will stabilize and a routine will emerge. Call on him, who is ever present, when you need to feel his peace. †

Never Be the Same

"Now the LORD *is the Spirit, and where the Spirit of the* LORD *is, there is freedom. And we, who with unveiled faces all reflect the* LORD*'s glory, are being transformed into his likeness with ever-increasing glory, which comes from the* LORD*, who is the Spirit."*

2 CORINTHIANS 3:17–19

Becoming a mother is a completely life-altering experience, challenging the perspective through which you've viewed your life thus far. For the first time, you'll probably begin to grasp how much your own parents love you. You will feel a sense of love and protection for another creature that will never change, regardless of age. Rather than making choices based on what you want, choices will be motivated by what's best for your family. You can never go back to the person you were before, because motherhood has changed you.

When we become Christians, it is much the same transformation. We are consumed with his grace for us, so thankful for the love he extends to us. When we reflect on our former ways, we shudder at how we used to live, recognizing how close we all were to the clutch of the enemy. As a believer in Christ, we will never be the same again. †

DAY 271

Thoroughly Equipped

"All Scripture is God-breathed and is useful for teaching, rebuking, correcting and training in righteousness, so that the man of God may be thoroughly equipped for every good work."

2 TIMOTHY 3:16–17

Your hospital bag is fully stocked with pajamas, camera, snacks, books, and clothes. You may have your cell phone ready to announce the good news, programmed with the numbers of everyone you know. Friends and family are calling regularly, asking for updates. Your home is stocked with diapers, a bassinet or crib for Baby, a swing, bottles, and more. You are fully equipped to have this baby.

Yet, you may still have lingering doubts over your emotional or spiritual equipment. Have you thought, "What if I'm not a good mom? What if I don't know what to do?" But God has equipped you to be this child's mother. Look to Scripture when you feel unsure; it provides peace when you are discouraged, it provides correction and guidelines when you get off track. You have the Word, the God-breathed message to you for any and every area of your life. With it, you are well equipped for motherhood. †

Extraordinary Moments

"Therefore, since we are receiving a kingdom that cannot be shaken, let us be thankful, and so worship God acceptably with reverence and awe. . . ."

HEBREWS 12:28

The last weeks of my twin pregnancy were spent behind hospital walls. For weeks I left my bed only for restroom breaks. To be wheeled to another room for a sonogram was like being allowed a walk in the park. Eventually, I was allowed to take short walks down a window-lined walkway suspended between two buildings. There I was able to glimpse what I had been missing: breathing fresh air, holding my kids' hands in the parking lot, driving around the neighborhood, participating in society. What had once been mundane and ordinary was now extraordinary.

Do you take your extraordinary faith for granted? We neglect to appreciate our freedom to worship and praise God. We lose that excited expectation of coming into his presence, feeling him move among his body of believers. His Word is so readily available, in numerous Scripture translations, countless Bible studies, and even on the Internet, that we forget to be in awe of the privilege and opportunity to read his words. Remind yourself of the extraordinary in the ordinary today. †

DAY 273

Just Average

"With this in mind, we constantly pray for you, that our God may count you worthy of his calling, and that by his power he may fulfill every good purpose of yours and every act prompted by your faith."

2 THESSALONIANS 1:11

There are plenty of statistics. Ninety-eight percent of all deliveries occur within two weeks of the due date. The average baby weighs seven and a half pounds and is twenty inches long. Yet, when it comes to you and your baby, those numbers don't mean anything. Even if your baby meets every "average" parameter, your child is far from average. Your child has been formed and made for an extraordinary life, a life with purpose, calling, and meaning.

Do you ever feel like you are living a "just average" life? Have you forgotten the distinguishing characteristics that define you? Don't settle for an average life. Just as God has purposed your child for great living, so has he purposed you. Allow this new chapter to rejuvenate your originality, your creativity. Put your God-given talents and skills to work for his purposes. †

DAY 274

Purposeful Plans

"Many are the plans in a man's heart, but it is the LORD*'s purpose that prevails."*

PROVERBS 19:21

You likely haven't anticipated a birthday this eagerly since you were five years old. Now it's nearly birthday time for your baby, and you're as antsy as a child again. If you are anything like me, you've probably tried the mind-over-matter approach. Maybe you've been telling yourself over and over, "I will go into labor. My water will break. I will have contractions." Despite all the mental effort, you find yourself still quite pregnant, leaving you feeling disappointed, frustrated, and probably a bit depressed.

Your reward is coming very soon. Joyfully anticipate your baby's birth in God's perfect timing. Rather than willing your body to meet your timetable, set your focus on God's will, trusting in his perfect timing. He knows how and when your labor will start, how long it will last, and when it will culminate in the birth of your child. Only he knows why tomorrow or the next day is better than today. †

DAY 275

High Achiever

"Be still before the Lord *and wait patiently for him. . . ."*
Psalm 37:7

For several weeks, my doctor had been telling me, "Anytime now!" She recited my effacement percentage and centimeter dilation as though they were perfect SAT scores. I felt like the labor high achiever. Surely those signs meant something, right? Certainly my excellent effacement and dilation meant that my labor was imminent. But as one week passed, and then the next, the report remained the same. "Anytime now!" Despite my stellar scores, I still was not in labor.

Whether or not the baby drops, you lose your plug, or your cervix is dilating, the signs don't necessarily mean labor is any further away than a woman's who has done all of those things. You could still find yourself in the delivery room tomorrow. Don't focus on what you have not yet accomplished, but what you will. Wait patiently for his timing. †

DAY 276

The Permanent Period

"A woman giving birth to a child has pain because her time has come; but when her baby is born she forgets the anguish because of her joy that a child is born into the world. So with you: Now is your time of grief, but I will see you again and you will rejoice, and no one will take away your joy."

JOHN 16:21–22

Why was I still using pads ten days after delivery? I felt like I had a permanent period. It was one of those parts of pregnancy that I had either overlooked in my reading or gone into complete denial about. The disposable panties, pads the size of encyclopedias, and the painful cramping of my uterus after giving birth were not highlights of my pregnancy experience. Make sure you stock your hospital bag with a supply of your own sanitary pads, which may be more comfortable than the product issued by the hospital. You might also consider restocking your underwear drawer with panties that are comfortable on your postpregnancy body.

The unpleasant physical aspects of pregnancy will soon be a pale memory in comparison to the lifetime of joy you'll share with this child. Christ tells us that it will be the same when we are reunited with him in his kingdom; the grief and grievances of our earthly life will fade away in the face of our joy. †

DAY 277

Why Isn't He Worried?

"Above all, love each other deeply, because love covers over a multitude of sins. Offer hospitality to one another without grumbling."

1 PETER 4:8–9

I called him with my hourly contraction count. "What do you think it means?" I excitedly asked. "I think it means you're not in labor." It wasn't what I wanted to hear. How could my husband go about his business so calmly, working, doing yard work, and watching television? I could go into labor any minute. Didn't he care?

Though we can't always tell, most husbands are as excited about labor and delivery as their wives. They look forward to the baby's grand entrance as well as the return of their nonpregnant, "normal" wife. Though he isn't fixated on labor pains, he is worried about getting to the hospital on time or falling short when you need him most. While these last moments feel very much about you and the baby, your husband has an integral role to play as well. Love him deeply and assure him of how much you value all he is doing for you and your expanding family. †

Toy Training

"Therefore, holy brothers, who share in the heavenly calling, fix your thoughts on Jesus, the apostle and high priest whom we confess."

HEBREWS 3:1

Are you tired of watching the clock, complaining about your misery and wondering, "When, when, WHEN?" It's a good time to take out the toys and practice. As easy as the car seat looked in the store, actually fastening it in the car can be tricky. Practice snapping and buckling so you won't have to figure it out while Baby waits (and wails!) nearby.

Have you mastered the art of stroller contraction? Despite the ease with which they collapse for the store attendant, the last thing you want to do is to spend an hour trying to figure it out before you take the baby for a walk. Practice pulling it out of the car, opening and closing it, and making adjustments. These things sound easier than they actually are.

Mastering the equipment not only prepares you for mothering, but it also keeps your mind from wandering to dark and depressing places. As you work on these tasks, pray over the items, causing them to be sources of comfort and rest for the baby to come. †

DAY 279

It's His Fault

"To the woman he said, 'I will greatly increase your pains in childbearing; with pain you will give birth to children. . . .'"

GENESIS 3:16

Every woman responds to labor pain differently. For me, no matter how hard my husband tried to massage my back, he just made me feel worse. The way he fixated his hand over my face while counting and breathing just made me angry and nauseous. I didn't want him to touch me or tell me how to push. It is common for laboring wives to decide their husband is the sole reason for their pain, crying out, "This is ALL YOUR FAULT. You did this to me!"

Of course, we know that it isn't their fault at all, but more precisely our own. Because we are daughters of Eve, and share her sinful attributes, we live with the consequences of pain in childbirth. God still loved Adam and Eve, but because he is wholly holy, there had to be judgment for sin. Yet even in judgment, he loved them and stayed with them. He will be with you, too, as you labor, strengthening you and guiding you every step of the way. †

DAY 280

The End. The Beginning

"Find rest, O my soul, in God alone; my hope comes from him."
PSALM 62:5

Congratulations, you've made it to the end! Labor could be minutes or days away, but after all your waiting, growing, and praying, the end is here. You've endured every stage of pregnancy from morning sickness to stretch marks. You've mastered baby gear, side sleeping, rushing to the bathroom, food aversions and cravings. Through every pang of worry, every pound, every kick, and every contraction, you've drawn closer to God.

Now he'll be your partner in parenting as you cross the finish line of pregnancy and enter the marathon of motherhood. He will guide you with his words, directing your steps as you trust in him, ensuring that you are protected at every turn. When you fall down, as we all do sometimes, he will be there to pick up the pieces. When you get off track, he will lead you back. You will never be alone. †